Friedrich M. Wurst (Ed.) ■ **New and Upcoming Markers of Alcohol Consumption**

Friedrich M. Wurst
(Editor)

New and Upcoming Markers of Alcohol Consumption

STEINKOPFF

Springer

Editor
Dr. Friedrich M. Wurst
Psychiatric University Hospital
Wilhelm-Klein-Strasse 27
CH-4025 Basel
Switzerland

ISBN-13: 978-3-642-96010-9 e-ISBN-13: 978-3-642-96008-6
DOI: 10.1007/978-3-642-96008-6

Die Deutsche Bibliothek – CIP-Einheitsaufnahme
A catalogue record for this publication is available from Die Deutsche Bibliothek

Steinkopff Verlag Darmstadt
a member of BertelsmannSpringer Science+Business Media GmbH
http://www.steinkopff.springer.de

Softcover reprint of the hardcover 1st edition 2001

Medical Editor: Dr. Maria Magdalene Nabbe
Production: Heinz J. Schäfer
Cover Design: Erich Kirchner, Heidelberg
Typesetting: Datenübernahme von den Autoren

SPIN: 10791564 80/7231-5 4 3 2 1 0 – Printed on acid-free paper

This book is dedicated

to my family

Preface

New and upcoming markers of alcohol consumption

The abstinence oriented treatment of people with alcohol problems requires efficient methods for monitoring alcohol abstinence.

It is an important step in clinical and forensic practice to integrate biological state markers with a reasonable time frame of detection and a high sensivity and specificity to control alcohol use in the sense of lapse or relapse.

Friedrich Martin Wurst contributes continuously excellent research data and has meritoriously joined the most prominent specialists of all over the world to focus on different aspects of alcohol markers. I hope that this book will motivate people in basic research as well as clinicians to gain more knowledge and develop methods to treat people with alcohol problems.

Dr. Dieter Ladewig
Professor of Psychiatry and
Addiction Medicine
Department of Psychiatry
University Basel

Basel, November 6th. 2000

Foreword of the editor

Increasingly sophisticated methods to measure health and its burden, in particular the DALY (Disability Adjusted Life Year), have helped to provide a more balanced conception of the needs and priorities in the area of health for both developing and developed countries.
Both in developing countries and in industrialised societies mental problems account for about 10% of lost healthy years in life. This is twice the number for malignant neoplasms. Furthermore 5 of the 10 leading causes of disability world-wide (major depression, schizophrenia, bipolar disorders, alcohol use, obsessive compulsive disorders) are mental problems. In 1990 there have been 288 million cases of alcohol related diseases, which is about 5 times the number of schizophrenia in that year (http://www.who.int/inf-fs/en/fact217.html).
Therefore, to monitor alcohol consumption in clinical as well as in forensic practice, occupational medicine, at court and for traffic safety and safety at workplaces biological state markers of high sensitivity and specificity, capable of monitoring those in treatment for alcohol dependence or poly-drug-abusers as well as social drinkers in risky situations (driving, workplaces) are required. They are a necessity e.g. to improve diagnosis, therapy outcome and quality of life of the patients, increase safety both at workplaces and in traffic, avoid harm to the unborn during pregnancy (fetal alcohol syndrome), reduce costs, by making therapy more effective and reduce productivity loss.
Furthermore neuropsychological impairment following alcoholisation, though blood ethanol concentration is zero, usually referred to as hangover state might play a crucial role in accidents.
Numerous tests and devices (including sweat patches and transdermal electronic alcohol sensors) for different body fluids and tissues have been developed and suggested to disclose (recent) alcohol consumption.
The known markers, however can not be considered to be satisfying with regard to sensitivity and specificity. Furthermore, they do not cover the whole time axis for alcohol intake – i.e. there is a gap with regard to alcohol consumption of between 1 day and 1–2 weeks, between short – and long-term markers like ethanol, methanol, and CDT, GGT or MCV respectively. These traditional markers are in many cases besides alcohol influenced by age, gender and a variety of substances and non-alcohol associated diseases.

This book, emerging from a symposium at the World Congress of Psychiatry in Hamburg 1999, in the first chapter gives an overview on both state and trait markers form a psychiatric perspective, whereas the following chapters highlight some – by far not all – of the promising newer markers of alcohol consumption.
It is my distinct pleasure to thank the authors for providing the manuscripts and those, who made the publication possible, namely Organon Germany, Organon Switzerland, GlaxoSmithKline Switzerland and Steinkopff Verlag.
May this book stimulate research and debate in the field.

Basel, May 2001 Friedrich Martin Wurst

Table of contents

Biological and genetic markers of alcoholism – a psychiatric perspective

Gabi Koller
Michael Soyka

Ludwig-Maximilians Universität München
Psychiatric Departement
Nußbaumstraße 7
80336 Munich

Phone: +49-89-5160 5744
FAX: +49-89-5160 5748
Email: Gabi.Koller@psy.med.uni-muenchen.de

Abstract

With respect to alcoholism the term "marker" often is used misleading. Generally, state markers of alcoholism must be differentiated from trait markers or markers of alcohol intoxication. Trait markers are hereditary, time independent factors. Trait markers persist during the whole time. For alcoholism a number of possible neurochemical and neurophysiological trait markers including the monoaminoxidase-B-activity in platelets, activity of adenylatcyclase, endocrine markers (cortisol, ACTH, prolactin), dopamin-beta-hydroxylase, evoked potentials (P 300) and ADH/ALDH genotypes have been proposed, but none of these markers has been firmly established. State markers are occuring during the phases of alcohol consumption. State markers such as blood alcohol concentration, CDT, GGT, ASAT, ALAT, MCV, HDL- and VDRL-cholesterol, and others are widely used for diagnosis and screening of alcoholics but both sensitivity and specifity are limited (Gjerde et al., 1988). Also except for MCV, pathologic findings are bound to a relatively fast biological turnover and return to normal values in abstinent patients. Some authors shown association markers for example HLA antigen, blood groups or transketolase.

Alcohol markers of special relevance for psychiatric diagnosis are reviewed in this paper.

Trait Markers

Platelet Adenylyl Cyclase

The activities of some platelet enymes have been proposed to reflect changes of enzymes found in the brain. The activity of platelet adenylyl cyclase after stimualtion with guanine nucleotide, cesium flouride, or prostaglandine E1 was reported to be decreased in in alcoholics (Valverius et al., 1988). This was not associated with age, race, smoking or illicit drugs and there was no significant correlation with the duration alcohol intake. Activity was also decreased in alcoholics who abstained from alcohol for one or two years. These results were later confirmed and at this time no difference was found between typ I and typ II alcoholics (Parsian et al., 1996). In 1998 marked state dependent changes of lymphocyte adenylyl cyclase activities have been demonstrated in alcohol dependents during detoxification (Pauly et al., 1999). To date the possible role of a trait marker platelet adenylyl cyclase is not entirely clear.

Platelet Monoamine Oxidase

Platelet monoamine oxidase is a mitochondrial enzyme involved in the breakdown of neuronal transmitters like noradrenaline, adrenaline, dopamine or serotonine. Two isoenzymes are known, MAO A and MAO B. Both are found in the central nervous system. Type A is involved in the metabolism of serotonin and norepinephrine and type B degrades phenylethylamine and benzylamine. Only the latter form can be found in platelets. The genes for MAO-A and MAO-B are located in the short arm of human X chromosome 8 (Xp 11.3). Over 50-fold variations of MAO-A and MAO-B activities have been shown in humans (Murphy et al., 1979).

Low platelet monoamine oxidase (MAO) activity in human alcoholics as compared to controls has been found in many studies (Faraj et al., 1987), (Wiberg et al., 1977). Some studies failed to show this effect (Giller et al., 1984), (Tabakoff et al., 1988). Since alcoholism is a very heterogenous disorder with multiple subgroups more recent studies have tried to link reduced MAO B activity in alcoholics with certain personality traits or family history of alcoholism. In some studies a reduced MAO B activity in alcoholics was associated with type II alcoholism (Cloninger, 1987), a subtype which associated with high heretability, early age of onset and severe social and legal consequences of alcoholism (Pandey et al., 1988), (von Knorring et al., 1991), but several studies found no association between reduced MAO B activity and type II alcoholism (Yates et al., 1990), (Parsian et al., 1996). Especially the possible association of reduced platelet MAO B activity and family history of alcoholism has attracted substantial attention in recent years. A reduced activity has also been shown in relatives of alcoholics. (Alexopoulos et al., 1983; Coursey et al., 1982; Devor et al., 1993). Rommelspacher et al (1994) found a significantly lower platelet MAO B activity in alcoholics with high novelty-seeking and impulsiveness scores as measured by the Tridimensional Personality Questionnaire but these findings also need further confirmation (Rommelspacher et al., 1994).

Our own data (Soyka et al. 2000) demonstrate that there is no significant difference in MAO activity both with and without ethanol inhibition between family history positive (FHP) and family history negative (FHN) alcoholics and healthy controls. Also there were no significant differences concerning MAO activity in patients with and without antisocial personality traits. The only significant difference was a lower percentage of inhibition of MAO activity with ethanol in patients compared to controls. The latter finding is consistent with previous studies as cited above.

Dopaminreceptorgenes

There are five distinct forms of dopaminreceptors (D1 - D5). Dopaminreceptors were also object of investigation in search of biological correlates for alcoholism (Bolos et al., 1990; Parsian et al., 1991).
Alcoholism has also been associated with a particular polymorphism in the A1 allele of the dopamine D2 receptor (DRD2) gene (Blum et al., 1990) (Noble et al., 1991), but subsequent studies have questioned this finding (Gejman et al., 1994), or questioned the specifity of this finding for alcoholism (Comings et al., 1991). The literature on this topic is very broad now (Sander et al., 1995). More recent studies showed negative results (Laruelle et al., 1998) (Lee et al., 1999; Sander et al., 1999).

Dopaminergic and catecholaminergic system

It was suggested that disturbances in the regulation of catecholamine neuromediation are involved in the mechanism of developing alcoholism. For example, rats preferring and avoiding alcohol exhibit different dopamine and cyclic nucleotide concentrations in the blood and show different activities of some enzymes in the brain. Genetically determined abnormalities of catecholamine neuromediation in the brain may contribute to an individuals alcohol consume (Anokhina et al., 1988).
Another study found demented alcoholics to have significantly reduced plasma dopamine-beta-hydroxylase activity compared with non-demented alcoholic or with a control group. (Lykouras et al., 1987).

ACTH, cortisol and prolactine

In chronic alcohol consumers blunted ACTH release after CRH exposure is known even when the person lives abstinent for several weeks. Waltman et al (1994) investigated the ACTH response in sons of alcohol dependent fathers in comparison with family history negative sons. Ethanol or placebo was ingested, CRH was administered, and plasma ACTH/cortisol levels were determined. Men with family history positive had lower peak ACTH response to CRH than did family history negative men In family history negative men, plasma ACTH response to CRH was blunted during the ethanol session compared to the placebo session. In contrast, family history positive men had similar ACTH responses to CRH during ethanol and placebo sessions. Family history positive and family history negative nonalcoholic men had different plasma ACTH responses following the administration of CRH (Waltman et al., 1994).

A naloxone challenge was performed with family history positive sons in comparison with family history negative sons. Family history-positive men had increased ACTH response to naloxone compared to 1) family history-positive women, 2) family history-negative men, and 3) family history-negative women. This finding suggests that nonalcoholic male offspring of alcohol-dependent men have altered endogenous opioid activity directed at hypothalamic corticotropin-releasing factor neurons (Wand et al., 1999).

In a study from 1994 a relationship between $ALDH_2$ and cortisol levels was object of investigation. Subjects with $ALDH_2$ alleles demonstrated significantly higher cortisol levels after alcohol consumption than subjects with the $ALDH_2$ deficient genotype, despite equivalent blood alcohol concentrations. One subject who was homozygous for $ALDH_2$ had extraordinarily high cortisol levels. These data are consistent with the hypothesis that asians with $ALDH_2$ alleles, who flush after drinking, experience more intense reactions to alcohol than nonflushing Asians with the $ALDH_2$ deficient genotype (Wall et al., 1994).

Only a few studies investigate the relationship between prolactin and alcoholism. One of these data suggest the presence of an enhanced dopaminergic inhibitory control of PRL secretion in 2 - 3 week abstinent alcoholics with normal menstrual cycles and normal circulating estrogen levels. In contrast, amenorrhea in abstinent alcoholics appears to be associated with an enhancement of PRL cell secretory activity (Vescovi and Coiro, 1997).

Tryptophan hydroxylase gene

Tryptophan hydroxylase (TPH) is the rate-limiting enzyme in the synthesis of serotonin. Low turnover rate of this monoamine neurotransmitter is associated with impaired impulse control.

Sons of alcoholic fathers, who have committed violent crimes, have very low CSF 5-HIAA concentrations. Vagal tone does not correlate significantly with CSF 5-HIAA but correlates with enhanced insulin secretion, which is most prominent in subjects with intermittent explosive disorder. A polymorphism of tryptophan hydroxylase (TPH) gene is associated with low CSF 5-HIAA and a history of suicide attempts (Virkkunen et al., 1995). (Nielsen et al., 1998).

Neuropsychology

Some studies were made comparing sons of alcohol dependent fathers with sons of non alchol dependent fathers. The comparison was made in measuring intelligence, personality values and motoric ability. Sons of alcohol dependent fathers showed special deficits in motoric as well as memory effects and eloquence (MA, 1989). Sons of alcohol dependent father show more neuroticism and more social problems. Sons of alcoholdependent fathers show also deficits in visual and auditorial cognition.

Sons of alcohol dependent fathers show less sensitivity to low dose alcohol consumption and feel themselves less drunken after low dose alcohol consumption. (Schuckit, 1985).

Electrophysiological markers

Electric potentials in the brain are dependent on genetical influence. Because of this the electoencephalography and event related potential was object of investigation in alcohol dependents and their sons.

Electroencephalography

The brain is influenced by alcohol consumption in different ways. This can be shown by the electroencephalography.
Studies with monozygotic and heterozygotic twins lead to a genetic compound in the genesis of alcoholism. The influence of alcohol intake on α activity in the encephalography is the same in monozygotic twins (Propping, 1977).
Another object of investigation was the differences in electrography between sons of alcohol dependent individuals and healthy controls.
Gabrielli et al (1982) found in sons of alcohol dependent individuals α waves with higher frequencies than in controls. (Gabrielli et al., 1982). But some authors failed to show these results.

Evoked Potentials

Evoked potentials is a technology which allows to investigate the reaction of the brain after a stimulus. One famous object of investigation was the measuring of the amplitude of P 3. P 3 is the amplitude of evoked potentials which occurs 300 - 600 ms (for example P300) after a stimulus.
Begleiter et al. showed alcohol depedent individuals have a significantly reduced P3 compound in comparison with a control group. This result is reproduced several times (Porjesz and Begleiter, 1981). Similar results were published by other groups (Preuss et al., 1999) (Patterson et al., 1987), (Pfefferbaum et al., 1991).
Differences between alcohol dependent individuals and controls were also found in other parts of evoked potentials. But all kind of differences in evoked potentials found in alcohol dependent individuals dissappear in abstinence. Only P3 is also found in alcohol dependent individuals with long term abstinence.
Out of this young men with a high risk developing alcohol dependency were investigated. It was shown that P3 amplitude is lower in young men with high risk developing alcohol dependence than in young men with low risk depending alcohol dependence (Begleiter et al., 1984), (Connor et al., 1987), (Whipple et al., 1991).
Several studies showed same results, but some authors failed to replicate these results. Some authors found a reduction of P3 under acute alcohol intake. Schuckit et al. reported that individuals with high risk of developing an alcohol dependence return faster to normal P3 amlitude after alcohol intake than individuals with low risk developing an alcohol dependence (Polich and Bloom, 1988), (Schuckit MA, 1988).

Alcoholmetabolizing enzymes

Alcoldehydrogenase (ADH_2 and $ALDH_3$) and aldehyddehydrogenase has extensively been studied by various groups. ALDH plays an important role as trait marker of alcoholism.

In the body ethanol is oxidated into acetaldehyde. Alcoholdehydrogenase is the main catalysator of this proccess. The alcoholdehydrogenase protein contains different subgroups. Five different genloci localized on chromosom 4 are involved in synthesis of the different subgroups. ADH_2 is an atypical isoenzyme with higher specific activity. ADH_2 is detected in 15 – 20 % of european poulation and in 85 – 90 % of japanese and chinese population.
As a next step acetaldehyd is oxidated into acetat. This step is catalyzed by aldehyddehydrogenase. Aldehyddehydrogenase is located mainly in the liver enzymes. Most common is an ALDH form, which is deficient of $ALDH_2$. This form is found in 50 % of chinese and japanese population. A possible reason for this ALDH form is a mutation at point 487 which changes glutaminacid with lysin. This form is called the $ALDH_2$ deficient isoenzyme. In patients with alcoholism and alcohol induced liver damage a lower rate of $ALDH_2$ deficient isoenzyme appears (Shibuya and Yoshida, 1988). Chao et al have shown $ALDH_2$ and $ALDH_2$ gene to be assotiated with high risk for developing alcoholism or an alcohol induced liver damage (Chao et al., 1994).

State Markers

Blood parameters

CDT

In 1976 first time a protein fraction in the cerebrospinal fluid was detected by a swedish group around H. Stibler (Stibler, 1991).
This protein fraction was identified by isoelectric focussing as transferrin.
Transferrin is a 80 KD glycoproteine. In combination with the transferrin receptor it transports iron into the cells. (de Jong G, 1990), (van Noort et al., 1994).
Transferrin is a member of a gene family containing lots of members. The sequence is localized at the long arm of chromosome 3. About 90 % of all transferrin is synthesized in the liver. A smaller part is synthesized in the brain .
Transferrin contains one polypeptide and two carbohydrate side chains. (van Noort WL, 1994). Transferrin contains 6 % carbohydrate. This is bound at the end of the c-terminal end of asperaginacid as complex chains. These chains are containing oligosaccharide-n-acetylglucosamin. They are linked to mannose, galactose and sialinacid (Heegaard et al., 1989). The isoelectric point is defined by sialinacid. By isoelectric focussing the number of bound sialinacidrests is detectable. There are up to 6 sialinacids at one carbohydrate chain. The isoelectric point is defined by the amount of sialinacidrests. The most common so called type C of Transferrin has the isoelectric point of 5.4. In europe 98 % of population are transferrin type C.
After chronic alcohol intake the isoelectric point of transferrin is changing from 5.4 to over 5.6. This is caused by a lower amount of sialinacids. The amount of carbohydrates is also decreased. This transferrin is called carbohydrate-deficient-transferrin (CDT).

Not very much is known about the mechanisms why high levels of alcohol consumption induce CDT levels.
As a possible mechanism ethanol or acetaldehyde induced changes in the Golgi-apparatus during transferrin-carbohydrate chain synthesis are shown (Ghosh and Lakshman, 1997; van Noort WL, 1994). Other authors describe in the serum of alcohol abusers downregulated activity of galactosyl or n-acetylglucosaminyl-transferase activity, which is further downregulated in vitro by further acetaldehyde. (Stibler and Borg, 1991)
Even when the exact pathomechanism is not known there are lots of clinical trials showing that elevated CDT levels are associated with high levels of alcohol consumption (Soyka, 1995).
It is shown that one time alcohol excess is not able to change CDT levels (Allen et al., 1994). Even a regular alcohol consumption of 60g ethanol per day is not able to change CDT levels. It is documented that alcohol intake of more than 80g per day during more than 7 days may cause elevated CDT levels (Storey et al., 1985).
Plasma half time of CDT is about 14 days. But not everybody can reach normal CDT levels after 14 days of alcohol abstinence. This depends also on CDT levels before alcohol abstinence (Stibler, 1991).
At the beginning CDT was detected by isoelectric focussing. Soon after the detection of CDT a much easier method was developed (Stibler et al., 1986). This method contains an anionchangechromatography followed by a radioimmunoassay. There are different kinds of commercial used tests for CDT. Some tests show CDT as Units per liter others show CDT as percentage of total transferrin.
Depending on what kind of measurement is used normal values of CDT are about 20 U/l for men, 26 U/L for women or over 6 % CDT of total transferrin (Lesch et al., 1996).
Specificity of CDT as a marker of alcoholism is higher than sensitivity. Reasons for high CDT levels without chronic alcohol consumption are for example primary biliary cirrhosis, carbohydrate-deficient-glycoproteine syndrome, pregnancy and functional disorders of the liver.
Specificity of CDT as a marker of chronic alcoholism is meant to be higher than sensitivity. Specificity was shown in most clinical trials to be over 90 %. Sensitivity is shown to be about 90 %, but in some studies also much lower sensitivity is shown (Soyka, 1995).
In our own patients sensitivity is about 93.6 %, specificity is about 94.1 % (Soyka, 1999).
Sensitivity in CDT measured as U/l is as high as sensitivity measured in % of total transferrin.
CDT is not correlated with other markers of chronic alcoholism as GGT or MCV. In most cases it is necessary to analyze CDT as well as GGT and MCV.
For CDT elevation a chronic alcohol consumption of 2 - 3 weeks is necessary. While for an increase of GGT and MCV regularly alcohol consumption of 4 - 8 weeks is documented.
In conclusion CDT is a helpful marker in therapy of chronic alcohol consumers, because relapses can be recognized very soon.
In patients showing unclear elevated liver enzymes or MCV levels CDT may be a helpful instrument for the diagnosis of alcoholism. Also in medical certificates for

vehicular accidents CDT may be a helpful marker. Elevated CDT levels do not prove alcoholism. But in patients without hepatopathy elevated CDT levels should lead to an alcohol history.

In our own recent results (not yet published) sensitivity of CDT is 55 % and specificity is 96 %. Object of investigation was the correlation between the alcoholism marker CDT and psychomotoric tests. For this the "Wiener Testsystem" was used. Correlation between the tests and CDT was not significant, probably because CDT is a state marker which shows an overview over alcohol consumption between 2 – 4 weeks before the test (Horak et al. / to be submitted).

MCV

Additional state markers of heavy drinking include a mean corpuscular volume value of over 96 μm^3. This is due to alcohol toxic damage of bone mark. Another possible reason is a deficit of absorbic acid in alcohol dependents. Elevation of the mean corpuscular volume may also be caused by structural changes of the hemoglobin by acetaldehyde (Sillanaukee P, 1993). Sensitivity and specificity of MCV is much lower than in GGT or CDT. Elevated MCV values usually return to normal within 2 - 3 month, because of the long half live of erythrocytes. MCV is not influenced by short time alcohol abstinence, so it is very important in diagnosis of alcoholism. False positive MCV values occur in persons with non alcohol toxic bone mark damage, non alcohol toxic liver damage, reticulocytosis, deficits of vitamin B 12 and folic acid as well as heavy nicotine consume (Table 2).

State markers of alcoholism	False positive parameter
CDT	primary biliary cirrhosis, other kind of liver dysfunction carbohydrate-deficient-glycoprotein-syndrome pregnancy
GGT	viral hepatitis autoimmunhepatitis, primary biliary cirrhosis, obstruction of the ductus choledochus, cholangitis, diabetes, obesity, right heart failure, pregnancy, pancreatits, intoxicatin with aflatoxine or tetrachlorinecharcoal, anabolics, barbiturates, psychopharmacological agents, thyreostatic, zytotatics and oral contraceptive intake
GOT	all kind of liver disease
GPT	all kind of liver disease
GLDH	all kind of liver disease
HDL-cholesterol and apolipoproteine	physical activity, barbiturate and benzodiazepine intake, low body weight

State markers of alcoholism	False positive parameter
MCV	non alcohol toxic destruction of bone mark, non-alcohol toxic destruction of the liver, reticulocytosis, vitamin B12 deficiency, ascorbic acid deficiency, nicotine abuse
blood and urinary β-hexoaminidase	all kind of liver disease, renal disease, strenuous physical activity, aspirin intake and heat stress

Table 2 State markers of alcoholism and false positive test results

HDL-Cholesterin and Apolipoprotein

Several laboratory abnormalities are associated with excessive alcohol consumption. HDL cholesterin and apolipoprotein I/II are specific and sensitive for chronic alcohol consumption.
A possible reason for elevated HDL levels is an increased activity of lipoproteinlipase caused by induction of enzymes in combination with MEOS and GGT (Clemens MR, 1986).
Probably there is an relationship between low dose alcohol consumption, elevated HDL cholesterin and lower risk of coronary heart disease.
There is a wide variety of studies showing different data about high alcohol consumption and apolipoprotein as well as HDL cholesterin. Most of these data demonstrate a relationship between alcohol intake and apolipoprotein and HDL cholesterin levels. (Taskinen MR, 1982), (Glueck CJ, 1981), (Dai WS, 1985).

Liver enzymes

Gamma-Glutamyltransferase (GGT)

One of the most frequently used tests is gamma glutamyl transferase (GGT). Elevated GGT levels are not only caused by damage of hepatic cells. In most cases elevated GGT levels are caused by enzyminduction. If liver cells are damaged too there is an elevation of other liver enzymes as glutamat-oxalacetat-transaminase (GOT), glutamat-pyruvat-transaminase (GPT) or glutamat dehydrogenase (GLDH). There are a number of drinking experiments for GOT which show that a daily alcohol consumption of 60g alcohol per day for over 3 weeks is not enouh to induce an elevation (Gilg 1995).
Across several studies sensitivity is shown to be about 50 - 90 %. Specificity is only about 70 %. Sensitivity in GGT is lower than in CDT.
Normal values are shown to be for women 4 – 18 U/l for men 6 - 28 U/l. Propably normal values of GGT are defined too high, because in the examined population was no exclusion of alcohol dependents (Kornhuber, Bachhaus 1989). Usually GGT levels normalize after 2 - 5 weeks of abstinence from alcohol.

There are lots of factors causing elevated GGT levels (Table 1). For example pharmaceutics like thyreostatics, zytostatics, anabolics, barbiturates, oral contraceptives anabolics. Elevated GGT levels are also caused by viral hepatitis, autoimmunehepatitis, cholestatic hepatopathy, pregnancy and toxins like aflatoxin.

GOT (ASAT)

There are other important results related to the usual liver function test such as SGOT but this tend not to change unless actual liver cell alterations have occured. Sensitivity for alcoholism can be increased by using the De Ritis- Quotient (GOT/GPT > 1 - 2).

Trait-markers	Platelet Monoamine Oxidase Platelet Monoamine Oxidase (MAO-B) Dopaminreceptorgene Dopaminbetahydroxylase Endocrine Parameters like ACTH, Cortisol, Prolactin, TSH, TRH Alcoholdehydrogenase (ADH_2 ADH_3) Aldehydehydrogenase ($ALDH_2$ $ALDH_3$) Adenylatcyclase Visual Event Related Potential (EEG ERP) Tryptophanhydroxylase (5-HIAA)
State- (or intoxication) markers	CDT (Carbohydrate-deficient transferrin) GGT (Gammaglutamyltransferase) GPT (Glutamic Pyruvat Transaminase) GOT (Glutamic Oxalacetic Acid) GLDH (Glutamic Dehydrogenase) MCV (Mean Corpuscular Volume) AP (Alkaline Phosphatase) Blood and Urinary β-Hexoaminidase HDL Cholesterine and Apolipoproteine Blood Ethanol Concentration Acetaldehyde Acetat Tetrahydroquinolines
Association-markers	Bloodgroups, (MMS-blood group) HLA-Antigenes Transketolase

Table 1 Possible state markers, trait markers and parameters associated with alcoholism

Differentiation of alcohol induced hepatitis and other hepatopathies can be made by the testing of the mitochondrial GOT (mGOT) in relationship to total GOT (mGOT/GOT total).

Sensitivity and specificity in GOT is found to be much lower than in CDT (Nilssen et al., 1992).

GPT (ALAT)

Elevated GPT levels are also an expression of unspecific liver cell alterations. Elevated GPT levels should be discussed in combination with the other liver enzymes.

GLDH

GLDH was shown to be correlated with necrosis of liver cells. While elevation of GLDH was demonstrated after short time alcohol consumption too, this finding is discussed controversial (Haffner HT, 1988), (Gödde HW, 1989).

Blood and urinary β-Hexosaminidase

β-Hexosaminidase is a liver enzyme. It is detected by isoelectric focussing or by immunoassy. Sensitivity is shown to be higher than in GGT or GOT. Alcohol consumption of 60g per day for over 14 days induces an elevation of serum β-Hexoaminidase but not urinary β-Hexoaminidase levels. (Hultberg B, 1991) (Karkkainen and Salaspuro, 1991). Abnormal values are also found in many other conditions including liver, renal and some other diseasese. Furthermore physical activity, aspirin intake and heat may all result in elevated urinary β-Hexoaminidase levels.

Conclusion

To date, CDT and GGT are the most promsing clinical laboratory markers for alcoholism and alcohol relapse. Future researches will focus on short term markers of alcohol intake but also on promising new genetic markers.

References

Alexopoulos, G. S., Lieberman, K. W., and Frances, R. J. (1983). Platelet MAO activity in alcoholic patients and their first-degree relatives. Am J Psychiatry 140, 1501-4.

Allen, J. P., Litten, R. Z., Anton, R. F., and Cross, G. M. (1994). Carbohydrate-deficient transferrin as a measure of immoderate drinking: remaining issues. Alcohol Clin Exp Res 18, 799-812.

Anokhina, I. P., Kogan, B. M., and Drozdov, A. Z. (1988). Disturbances in regulation of catecholamine neuromediation in alcoholism. Alcohol Alcohol 23, 343-50.

Begleiter, H., Porjesz, B., Bihari, B., and Kissin, B. (1984). Event-related brain potentials in boys at risk for alcoholism. Science 225, 1493-6.

Blum, K., Noble, E. P., Sheridan, P. J., Montgomery, A., Ritchie, T., Jagadeeswaran, P., Nogami, H., Briggs, A. H., and Cohn, J. B. (1990). Allelic association of human dopamine D2 receptor gene in alcoholism [see comments]. Jama 263, 2055-60.

Bolos, A. M., Dean, M., Lucas Derse, S., Ramsburg, M., Brown, G. L., and Goldman, D. (1990). Population and pedigree studies reveal a lack of association between the dopamine D2 receptor gene and alcoholism [see comments]. Jama 264, 3156-60.

Chao, Y. C., Liou, S. R., Chung, Y. Y., Tang, H. S., Hsu, C. T., Li, T. K., and Yin, S. J. (1994). Polymorphism of alcohol and aldehyde dehydrogenase genes and alcoholic cirrhosis in Chinese patients. Hepatology 19, 360-6.

Clemens MR, S. H., Waller HD, (1986). Serumlipide von Alkoholikern vor und nach Abstinenz: Bedeutung für das Koronarrisiko. L Clin Chem Clin Biochem 24, 369-374.

Cloninger, C. R. (1987). Neurogenetic adaptive mechanisms in alcoholism. Science 236, 410-6.

Comings, D. E., Comings, B. G., Muhleman, D., Dietz, G., Shahbahrami, B., Tast, D., Knell, E., Kocsis, P., Baumgarten, R., Kovacs, B. W., and et al. (1991). The dopamine D2 receptor locus as a modifying gene in neuropsychiatric disorders [see comments]. Jama 266, 1793-800.

Connor, S. O., Hesselbrock, V., Tasman, A., and DePalma, N. (1987). P3 amplitudes in two distinct tasks are decreased in young men with a history of paternal alcoholism. Alcohol 4, 323-30.

Coursey, R. D., Buchsbaum, M. S., and Murphy, D. L. (1982). 2-year follow-up of subjects and their families defined as at risk for psychopathology on the basis of platelet MAO activities. 2-year follow-up of low platelet MAO. Neuropsychobiology 8, 51-6.

Dai WS, L. R., Hom DL et al (1985). Alcohol Consumption and High Density Lipoprotein Cholesterol Concentration Among Alcoholics. Am J of Epidemiol 122, 620-628.

De Jong G, v. D. J., van Eijk HG, (1990). The biology of transferrin. Clin Chim Acta 190, 1-46.

Devor, E. J., Cloninger, C. R., Kwan, S. W., and Abell, C. W. (1993). A genetic familial study of monoamine oxidase B activity and concentration in alcoholics. Alcohol Clin Exp Res 17, 263-7.

Faraj, B. A., Lenton, J. D., Kutner, M., Camp, V. M., Stammers, T. W., Lee, S. R., Lolies, P. A., and Chandora, D. (1987). Prevalence of low monoamine oxidase function in alcoholism. Alcohol Clin Exp Res 11, 464-7.

Gabrielli, W. F., Jr., Mednick, S. A., Volavka, J., Pollock, V. E., Schulsinger, F., and Itil, T. M. (1982). Electroencephalograms in children of alcoholic fathers. Psychophysiology 19, 404-7.

Gejman, P. V., Ram, A., Gelernter, J., Friedman, E., Cao, Q., Pickar, D., Blum, K., Noble, E. P., Kranzler, H. R., S, O. M., and et al. (1994). No structural mutation in the dopamine D2 receptor gene in alcoholism or schizophrenia. Analysis using denaturing gradient gel electrophoresis. Jama 271, 204-8.

Ghosh, P., and Lakshman, M. R. (1997). Chronic ethanol induced impairment of hepatic glycosylation machinery in rat is independent of dietary carbohydrate. Alcohol Clin Exp Res 21, 76-81.

Giller, E., Jr., Nocks, J., Hall, H., Stewart, C., Schnitt, J., and Sherman, B. (1984). Platelet and fibroblast monoamine oxidase in alcoholism. Psychiatry Res 12, 339-47.

Gjerde, H., Johnsen, J., Bjorneboe, A., Bjorneboe, G. E., and Morland, J. (1988). A comparison of serum carbohydrate-deficient transferrin with other biological markers of excessive drinking. Scand J Clin Lab Invest 48, 1-6.

Glueck CJ, H. G., Morrison JA, Khoury P, Moore M (1981). Alcohol intake, cigarette smoking and plasma lipidsm and Lipoproteins in 12-19 year old Children. Circulation 64, 48-56.

Gödde HW, A. D. (1989). Alcoholism: Biomedical and genetic aspects. Pergamon Press.

Haffner HT, K. M., Zink P (1988). Veränderung der Leberenzyme im Verlauf einer 36stündigen Alkoholbelastung. Blutalkohol 25, 116-126.

Heegaard, N. H., Hagerup, M., Thomsen, A. C., and Heegaard, P. M. (1989). Concanavalin A crossed affinity immunoelectrophoresis and image analysis for semiquantitative evaluation of microhete-

rogeneity profiles of human serum transferrin from alcoholics and normal individuals. Electrophoresis 10, 836-40.
Hultberg B, I. A., Berglund M, Moberg AL, (1991). Serum beta-hexoaminidase isoenzyme: a sensitive marker for alcohol abuse. Alcohol Clin Ex Res 15, 549-5521.
Karkkainen, P., and Salaspuro, M. (1991). beta-Hexosaminidase in the detection of alcoholism and heavy drinking. Alcohol Alcohol Suppl 1, 459-64.
Laruelle, M., Gelernter, J., and Innis, R. B. (1998). D2 receptors binding potential is not affected by Taq1 polymorphism at the D2 receptor gene. Mol Psychiatry 3, 261-5.
Lee, J. F., Lu, R. B., Ko, H. C., Chang, F. M., Yin, S. J., Pakstis, A. J., and Kidd, K. K. (1999). No association between DRD2 locus and alcoholism after controlling the ADH and ALDH genotypes in Chinese Han population. Alcohol Clin Exp Res 23, 592-9.
Lesch, O. M., Walter, H., Antal, J., Heggli, D. E., Kovacz, A., Leitner, A., Neumeister, A., Stumpf, I., Sundrehagen, E., and Kasper, S. (1996). Carbohydrate-deficient transferrin as a marker of alcohol intake: a study with healthy subjects. Alcohol Alcohol 31, 265-71.
Lykouras, E., Moussas, G., and Markianos, M. (1987). Platelet monoamine oxidase and plasma dopamine-beta-hydroxylase activities in non-abstinent chronic alcoholics. Relation to clinical parameters. Drug Alcohol Depend 19, 363-8.
MA, S. (1989). Biomedical and genetic markers of alcoholism. Goedde HW, Agarwl DP, Alcoholism: biomedical and genetic aspects, 290-302.
Murphy, D. L., Redmond, D. E., Jr., Garrick, N., and Baulu, J. (1979). Brain region differences and some characteristics of monoamine oxidase type A and B activities in the vervet monkey. Neurochem Res 4, 53-62.
Nielsen, D. A., Virkkunen, M., Lappalainen, J., Eggert, M., Brown, G. L., Long, J. C., Goldman, D., and Linnoila, M. (1998). A tryptophan hydroxylase gene marker for suicidality and alcoholism. Arch Gen Psychiatry 55, 593-602.
Nilssen, O., Huseby, N. E., Hoyer, G., Brenn, T., Schirmer, H., and Forde, O. H. (1992). New alcohol markers--how useful are they in population studies: the Svalbard Study 1988-89. Alcohol Clin Exp Res 16, 82-6.
Noble, E. P., Blum, K., Ritchie, T., Montgomery, A., and Sheridan, P. J. (1991). Allelic association of the D2 dopamine receptor gene with receptor-binding characteristics in alcoholism. Arch Gen Psychiatry 48, 648-54.
Pandey, G. N., Fawcett, J., Gibbons, R., Clark, D. C., and Davis, J. M. (1988). Platelet monoamine oxidase in alcoholism. Biol Psychiatry 24, 15-24.
Parsian, A., Todd, R. D., Cloninger, C. R., Hoffman, P. L., Ovchinnikova, L., Ikeda, H., and Tabakoff, B. (1996). Platelet adenylyl cyclase activity in alcoholics and subtypes of alcoholics. WHO/ISBRA Study Clinical Centers. Alcohol Clin Exp Res 20, 745-51.
Parsian, A., Todd, R. D., Devor, E. J., KL, O. M., Suarez, B. K., Reich, T., and Cloninger, C. R. (1991). Alcoholism and alleles of the human D2 dopamine receptor locus. Studies of association and linkage. Arch Gen Psychiatry 48, 655-63.
Patterson, B. W., Williams, H. L., McLean, G. A., Smith, L. T., and Schaeffer, K. W. (1987). Alcoholism and family history of alcoholism: effects on visual and auditory event-related potentials. Alcohol 4, 265-74.
Pauly, T., Dahmen, N., Szegedi, A., Wetzel, H., Bol, G. F., Ferdinand, K., and Hiemke, C. (1999). Blood ethanol levels and adenylyl cyclase activity in lymphocytes of alcoholic patients. Biol Psychiatry 45, 489-93.
Pfefferbaum, A., Ford, J. M., White, P. M., and Mathalon, D. (1991). Event-related potentials in alcoholic men: P3 amplitude reflects family history but not alcohol consumption. Alcohol Clin Exp Res 15, 839-50.
Polich, J., and Bloom, F. E. (1988). Event-related brain potentials in individuals at high and low risk for developing alcoholism: failure to replicate. Alcohol Clin Exp Res 12, 368-73.
Porjesz, B., and Begleiter, H. (1981). Human evoked brain potentials and alcohol. Alcohol Clin Exp Res 5, 304-17.
Preuss, U. W., Frodl Bauch, T., Benda, E., Soyka, M., Moller, H., and Hegerl, U. (1999). Late auditory evoked potentials (P300) do not discriminate between subgroups of alcohol-dependent patients defined by family history and antisocial personality traits. Eur J Med Res 4, 114-20.
Propping, P. (1977). Genetic control of ethanol action on the central nervous system. An EEG study in twins. Hum Genet 35, 309-34.

Rommelspacher, H., May, T., Dufeu, P., and Schmidt, L. G. (1994). Longitudinal observations of monoamine oxidase B in alcoholics: differentiation of marker characteristics. Alcohol Clin Exp Res 18, 1322-9.

Sander, T., Harms, H., Podschus, J., Finckh, U., Nickel, B., Rolfs, A., Rommelspacher, H., and Schmidt, L. G. (1995). Dopamine D1, D2 and D3 receptor genes in alcohol dependence. Psychiatr Genet 5, 171-6.

Sander, T., Ladehoff, M., Samochowiec, J., Finckh, U., Rommelspacher, H., and Schmidt, L. G. (1999). Lack of an allelic association between polymorphisms of the dopamine D2 receptor gene and alcohol dependence in the German population. Alcohol Clin Exp Res 23, 578-81.

Schuckit, M. A. (1985). Ethanol-induced changes in body sway in men at high alcoholism risk. Arch Gen Psychiatry 42, 375-9.

Schuckit MA, I. M., Monteiro MG, (1988). Differences in intensity of Reaction to Ethanol in Children of Alcoholics and Controls. Proceedings of 4th ISBRA Congres, Kyoto, 453-457.

Shibuya, A., and Yoshida, A. (1988). Genotypes of alcohol-metabolizing enzymes in Japanese with alcohol liver diseases: a strong association of the usual Caucasian-type aldehyde dehydrogenase gene (ALDH1(2)) with the disease [published erratum appears in Am J Hum Genet 1989 Apr;44(4):619]. Am J Hum Genet 43, 744-8.

Sillanaukee P, S. K., Koivula T, (1993). Effect ofacetaldhyde on hemoglobin: HbA1c act as a potential marker of heavy drinking. Alcohol 8, 377-381.

Soyka, M. (1995). Die Alkoholkrankheit-Diagnostik und Therapie (Weinheim: Chapman&Hall).

Soyka, M. (1999). Klinische Alkoholismusdiagnostik, Steinkopff, ed. (Darmstadt: Soyka, M).

Soyka, M., Bondy, B., Benda, E., Preuss, U., Hegerl, U., Möller, H. J.. Platelet monoamine, oxidase activity in alcoholics with and without a histroy of alcoholism. Euv Addict Res. 6, 57-63 (2000)

Stibler, H. (1991). Carbohydrate-deficient transferrin in serum: a new marker of potentially harmful alcohol consumption reviewed. Clin Chem 37, 2029-37.

Stibler, H., and Borg, S. (1991). Glycoprotein glycosyltransferase activities in serum in alcohol-abusing patients and healthy controls. Scand J Clin Lab Invest 51, 43-51.

Stibler, H., Borg, S., and Joustra, M. (1986). Micro anion exchange chromatography of carbohydrate-deficient transferrin in serum in relation to alcohol consumption (Swedish Patent 8400587-5). Alcohol Clin Exp Res 10, 535-44.

Storey, E. L., Mack, U., Powell, L. W., and Halliday, J. W. (1985). Use of chromatofocusing to detect a transferrin variant in serum of alcoholic subjects. Clin Chem 31, 1543-5.

Tabakoff, B., Hoffman, P. L., Lee, J. M., Saito, T., Willard, B., and De Leon Jones, F. (1988). Differences in platelet enzyme activity between alcoholics and nonalcoholics. N Engl J Med 318, 134-9.

Taskinen MR, V. M., Nikkilä EA et al. (1982). High density lipoprotein subfractions and postheparin plasma lipases in alcoholic men before and after alcohol withdrawal. Metaboilsm 31, 1168-1171.

Valverius, P., Hoffman, P. L., and Tabakoff, B. (1988). Effects of chronic ethanol ingestion on mouse brain beta-adrenergic receptors (BAR) and adenylate cyclase. Adv Alcohol Subst Abuse 7, 99-101.

Van Noort, W. L., de Jong, G., and van Eijk, H. G. (1994). Purification of isotransferrins by concanavalin A sepharose chromatography and preparative isoelectric focusing. Eur J Clin Chem Clin Biochem 32, 885-92.

Van Noort WL, d. J. G., van Eijk HG, (1994). Purification of isotransferrins by concanavalin. A sepharose chromatographie and preparative isoelectric focussing. Eur J of Clin Chem Clin Biochem 32, 885-892.

Vescovi, P. P., and Coiro, V. (1997). Effects of thyrotropin-releasing hormone and metoclopramide on PRL secretion in normally cycling and amenorrheic alcoholic women. Drug Alcohol Depend 45, 115-9.

Virkkunen, M., Goldman, D., Nielsen, D. A., and Linnoila, M. (1995). Low brain serotonin turnover rate (low CSF 5-HIAA) and impulsive violence. J Psychiatry Neurosci 20, 271-5.

Von Knorring, A. L., Hallman, J., von Knorring, L., and Oreland, L. (1991). Platelet monoamine oxidase activity in type 1 and type 2 alcoholism. Alcohol Alcohol 26, 409-16.

Wall, T. L., Nemeroff, C. B., Ritchie, J. C., and Ehlers, C. L. (1994). Cortisol responses following placebo and alcohol in Asians with different ALDH2 genotypes. J Stud Alcohol 55, 207-13.

Waltman, C., McCaul, M. E., and Wand, G. S. (1994). Adrenocorticotropin responses following administration of ethanol and ovine corticotropin-releasing hormone in the sons of alcoholics and control subjects. Alcohol Clin Exp Res 18, 826-30.

Wand, G. S., Mangold, D., and Ali, M. (1999). Adrenocorticotropin responses to naloxone in sons of alcohol-dependent men. J Clin Endocrinol Metab 84, 64-8.

Whipple, S. C., Berman, S. M., and Noble, E. P. (1991). Event-related potentials in alcoholic fathers and their sons. Alcohol 8, 321-7.
Wiberg, A., Wahlstroom, G., and Oreland, L. (1977). Brain monoamine oxidase activity after chronic ethanol treatment of rats. Psychopharmacology Berl 52, 111-3.
Yates, W. R., Wilcox, J., Knudson, R., Myers, C., and Kelly, M. W. (1990). The effect of gender and subtype on platelet MAO in alcoholism. J Stud Alcohol 51, 463-7.

Possible role of long chain fatty acid ethyl esters in organ injury and as short-term markers of ethanol intake in humans

Margareta A. Diczfalusy
Mats von Wachenfeldt
Inger Holmberg
Stefan E.H. Alexson

Department of Medical Laboratory Sciences and Technology, Division of Clinical Chemistry, Department of Surgery and Department of Internal Medicine, Division of Gastroenterology and Hepatology, Karolinska Institute, Huddinge University Hospital, S-141 86 Huddinge, Sweden

Address for correspondence:
Stefan Alexson
Department of Medical Laboratory Sciences and Technology
Division of Clinical Chemistry
Karolinska Institutet
Huddinge University Hospital
S-141 86 Huddinge
Sweden

Phone: +46-8-5858 1274
FAX: +46-8-5858 1260
Email: stefan.alexson@chemlab.hs.sll.se

Abbreviations
AEAT, acyl-coenzyme A:ethanol *O*-acyltransferase; FAEE, fatty acid ethyl ester; ES-4 and ES-10, rat liver microsomal carboxylesterases; BNPP, bis-(4-nitrophenyl) phosphate; p-HMB, p-hydroxymercuribenzoic acid.

Abstract

Ingested ethanol is mainly oxidized to acetaldehyde and acetate in the liver and oxidative metabolites of ethanol have been implicated in organ injury. More recently, fatty acid ethyl esters (FAEEs), non-oxidative metabolites of ethanol, have been shown to be present in blood and in a number of organs with low or no capacity to oxidize ethanol, after alcohol intake. As such esters may have detrimental effects on subcellular structures, they have been proposed as possible mediators of injury in organs lacking oxidative ethanol metabolism. Two enzyme activities, acyl-CoA; ethanol *O*-acyltransferase (AEAT) and fatty acid ethyl ester (FAEE) synthase have the ability to esterify fatty acids to ethanol. We have characterized these two activities in rat and human liver microsomes and measured the activities in various human organs. Our data strongly suggest that AEAT is of major importance for the formation of FAEEs both in rat and in humans. Of the human tissues tested, liver had the clearly highest FAEE-synthesizing activity, but high activity was also found in intestinal mucosa. Pancreas contained relatively low capacity to synthesize FAEEs (with AEAT and FAEE synthase activities being comparable). Liver and pancreas contained very high FAEE hydrolyzing activity, while it was very low in intestine. Considering the central role of the intestine in uptake and esterification of fatty acids, and uptake of ingested alcohol, intestine is likely to be an important site for the synthsis of FAEEs. In addition, human serum contains very low FAEE hydrolyzing activity which can account for the observed elevation of FAEEs in blood during alcohol intake. In a controlled alcohol intake experiment we found that FAEEs appeared rapidly in the blood, with increased levels being detectable several hours after disappearence of blood ethanol. These data suggest that FAEEs may be used as a short term marker for ethanol intake.

Introduction

Ethanol is mainly metabolized by oxidation to acetaldehyde and acetate in the liver. The oxidation of ethanol is catalyzed by three classes of enzymes, by alcohol dehydrogenases (localized in the cytosol) which account for the major oxidative pathway, by catalase present in peroxisomes and by cytochrome P-450 IIE1 located in the endoplasmic reticulum, for review see (Lieber, 1985). Catalase and the microsomal P-450 IIE1 are of minor importance during normal conditions. Acetaldehyde is further oxidized to acetate by acetaldehyde dehydrogenase, followed by oxidation to CO_2 and water in peripheral tissues. Several pathological consequences of alcohol abuse have been attributed to products generated by the oxidative pathways, i.e. acetaldehyde and acetate, due to their interactions with various metabolic functions. However, several organs with a limited capacity to oxidize ethanol, such as heart, pancreas and brain, are also injured in alcoholics. Furthermore, acetaldehyde which is primarily generated in the liver has been found in negligible concentrations in the circulation after ethanol intake. These findings suggest that other factors than oxidative metabolites of ethanol may be responsible for ethanol-induced injury in organs lacking oxidative ethanol metabolism. More recently fatty acid esters of ethanol (FAEEs) have been implicated as possible mediators of at least some of the toxic effects associated with alcohol consumption. Post-mortem analysis of lipids in organs showed that FAEEs could be detected in several organs of "social drinkers", and that elevated concentrations of FAEEs could be detected in patients acutely intoxicated with ethanol compared to non-alcohol drinking subjects (Laposata and Lange, 1986). Also occurrence of FAEEs in serum of subjects participating in controlled ethanol ingestion studies have been demonstrated, with changes in the levels closely correlating with changes in the concentration of serum ethanol (Doyle, et al., 1996; Dan and Laposata, 1997; Soderberg, et al., 1999).

There is still no evidence that FAEEs are involved in organ injury and the possible mechanisms are not known. However, FAEEs have been shown to e.g. uncouple mitochondrial phosphorylation in rabbit heart (Lange and Sobel, 1983), inhibit protein synthesis and cell proliferation in human hepatoblastoma cells (Szczypiorkowski, et al., 1995) and increase fragility of pancreatic lysosomes (Haber, et al., 1993). Although FAEEs seem to be present in various human tissues, there is still only limited knowledge about the biochemical origin of FAEEs in these tissues. FAEEs found in human tissues may be derived from local synthesis, or synthesized in other tissues or blood and delivered via the circulation to various organs. In addition accumulation of FAEEs in various organs is probably dependent on the capacity of various tissues to hydrolyze FAEEs.

There are two enzymatic activities catalyzing the formation of FAEEs: acyl-coenzyme A:ethanol *O*-acyltransferase (AEAT) and fatty acid ethyl ester (FAEE) synthase. FAEE synthases have been purified from several sources such as rabbit myocardium, human brain and rat adipose tissue and two of these FAEE synthases were found to be identical to rat liver carboxylesterase (Tsujita and Okuda, 1992; Bora, et al., 1996). Furthermore, a variety of other enzymes such as e.g. pancreatic lipase, lipoprotein lipase and glutathione transferases have been shown to possess FAEE synthase activity (Tsujita and Okuda, 1992; Bora, et al., 1989; Riley, et al., 1990; Tsujita and Okuda, 1994; Chang, et al., 1997). At present there is no evidence for the existence of a specific FAEE synthase and the formation of FAEEs from free fatty acids seems to be a result of the action of several enzymes with other functions. The enzyme responsible for most of the AEAT activity in rat liver is localized at the lumenal side of the endoplasmic reticulum (Polokoff and Bell, 1978), but has not yet been identified or purified. Characterization of AEAT and FAEE synthase activities using isolated rat liver microsomes suggests that AEAT is quantitatively the most important of these two activities (Diczfalusy, et al., 1999). Still, however, conclusive evidence for the involvement of FAEEs in organ injury is lacking and the relative significance of AEAT and FAEE synthase for the formation of FAEEs in humans has not yet been elucidated. We here summarize our experiments on the biochemical characterization of the enzymes involved in formation of FAEEs in rat and human. We also show that FAEEs can be detected in blood during controlled ethanol intake and that FAEEs remain elevated in serum for some time after disappearence of blood ethanol, suggesting that FAEEs may be used as a short-term marker for ethanol intake.

Materials and methods

Animals

Sprague-Dawley rats weighing about 200 g were obtained from B&K Universal AB (Sollentuna, Sweden). The rats were fed standard rat chow and had access to water ad libitum. The rats were euthanized with CO_2 and blood was collected by heart puncture. Serum was prepared by centrifugation of blood samples at 2700 rpm for 15 minutes. The livers were dissected out and immediately chilled in ice-cold sucrose medium (0.25 M sucrose, 10 mM Tris-HCl, 1 mM EDTA, 0.1 % ethanol, pH 7.4).

Patients and tissue sampling

Tissues were obtained from 17 patients undergoing elective surgery. Peroperative liver biopsies, for preparation of microsomes, were obtained from patients undergoing cholecystectomy. Gall-bladder samples were obtained from patients operated for uncomplicated gallstone disease. Normal tissue of the pancreatic head and biopsies from adipose tissue were obtained from patients undergoing Whipple resection due to cholangiocarcinoma of the lower bile duct. Normal lung tissue was from patients operated for lung cancer. Heart muscle tissue was obtained from the auricle of the right atrium of patients undergoing coronary by-pass operation. Samples of normal small intestine were obtained from two patients undergoing pancreaticoduodenectomy by Whipple resection because of carcinoma of the pancreatic head and carcinoma of the bile duct, respectively. The tissues were immediately frozen and stored in liquid nitrogen until analysis. Informed consent was obtained from each patient before the operation, and the ethical aspects of the study were approved by the Ethical Committee at Karolinska Institute, Stockholm.

Preparation of tissue homogenates and isolation of liver microsomes

The frozen tissues were thawed, minced and homogenized with a loose fitting pestle in nine volumes of ice-cold 50 mM potassium phosphate buffer containing 0.5 mM EDTA (pH 7.4). The homogenates were filtered through a double layer of gauze and stored at –20 ^{0}C in aliquots.

Liver microsomes were prepared as described earlier (Einarsson, et al., 1989), and the resulting microsomal pellet was suspended in 100 mM potassium phosphate buffer containing 1 mM EDTA (pH 7.4) and stored at -20 ^{0}C in aliquots. Protein was determined by the method of Bradford, using bovine serum albumin as standard (Bradford, 1976).

AEAT assay

AEAT activity was measured as described earlier (Diczfalusy, et al., 1999). Briefly, 100 μM [1-14C]palmitoyl-CoA, 0.86 M ethanol, 2 mg/ml HSA, 250 μM bis(4-nitrophenyl) phosphate (BNPP) and enzyme (5 - 10 μg of microsomal protein or 10 - 72 μg of tissue homogenate protein) were preincubated for 20 minutes at 37^{0}C in 100 mM potassium phosphate buffer, 1 mM EDTA, pH 7.4, in a total volume 0.25 ml. The reaction was started by addition of the substrates (ethanol and [1-14C]palmitoyl-CoA) and incubated for about 15 minutes and the reaction was stopped by addition of 1.6 ml ice-cold heptane. Ethyl palmitate was extracted with heptane as described earlier (Polokoff and Bell, 1978), with minor modifications (Diczfalusy, et al., 1999). Blank incubations, containing all components except enzyme, were run in parallel. The product was quantitated by liquid scintillation counting of 0.8 ml of the heptane phase, and AEAT activity, corrected for the blanks, was expressed as nanomoles of [14C]ethyl palmitate formed per minute and milligram of microsomal protein, or per minute and gram tissue when measured in homogenates.

FAEE synthase assay

About 50 μg of microsomal protein or tissue homogenate protein was preincubated for 15 minutes at 37^{0}C in 100 mM potassium phosphate buffer containing 1 mM EDTA (pH 7.4), and the reaction was started by addition of 0.4 mM [1-14C]palmitic acid and 0.86 M ethanol. The total incubation volume was 0.25 ml. The reaction was stopped after 20 minutes by addition of 1.6 ml of ice-cold heptane and ethyl palmitate was extracted and quantitated as described above for determination of AEAT activity.

Hydrolysis of [14C]ethyl palmitate

About 2 μg of microsomal protein, or 20 - 60 μg of tissue homogenate protein, was preincubated in 100 mM potassium phosphate buffer (pH 7.4) containing 1 mM EDTA and 2 mg/mL HSA in a total volume of 0.25 ml for 20 min at 37^{0}C. The reaction was started by addition of 0.175 mM [14C]ethyl palmitate (synthesized from [1-14C] palmitic acid and ethanol as described previously (Diczfalusy, et al., 1999) and the samples were incubated for about 15 minutes. The incubation was terminated by addition of 2.5 ml chloroform/methanol (2:1, v/v) and 250 µl of 0.1 M H_2SO_4 in 0.9 % NaCl. The chloroform phase was evaporated under reduced pressure and the radioactive lipids were dissolved in a small volume of chloroform/methanol (2:1, v/v) and chromatographed on Silica Gel 60 plates developed in hexane:diethyl ether:glacial acetic acid, 80:20:1 (v/v/v). The TLC plates were scannned for radioactivity and the spots corresponding to [14C]ethyl palmitate and [14C]palmitic acid were scraped off and counted in a liquid scintillation counter.

Formation of FAEE in vivo

One apparently healthy volunter (fasted overnight) of the laboratory staff received 160 ml of an alcoholic beverage (40 % ethanol). The alcoholic beverage was divided into four aliquots of 40 ml which were administered orally every 15 minutes for a total drinking period of 45 min. Blood samples were drawn at 0, 30, 60, 90, 120, 150, 190, 240, 300 and 360 minutes after the ethanol intake via a saline-flushed catheter. An additional blood sample was obtained 24 h after the start of the experiment. A meal was served 240 min after administration of the first aliquot of alcoholic beverage. The blood samples were collected in vacuum tubes without anticoagulant and sera were prepared by centrifugation at 1250 x g for 10 min and stored in 1 ml aliquots at -70^{0}C. Blood ethanol was determined by a routine method at the Division of Clinical Chemistry, Huddinge University Hospital.

Solid-phase extraction of FAEEs from sera and gas chromatography (GC)

Lipids were extracted from i ml serum by addition of 2 ml of acetone, followed by addition of 5 ml of hexane and 800 ng (dissolved in 80 µl of ethanol) of an internal standard [nonadecanoic (C19:0) acid etyl ester]. After vortex mixing for 1 min, the samples were centrifuged at 175 x g for 5 min and the hexane-acetone phase was transferred to a separate tube, evaporated to dryness under nitrogen, resuspended in 200 µl of hexane and applied to an aminopropyl-silica column. The column was pre-washed with hexane and the sample was applied to the column and eluted with 4 ml of hexane. The hexane eluate was then evaporated under nitrogen and resuspended in 100 µl of hexane out of which 2 µl was subjected to GC analysis. GC analysis was performed using a HP 5890 gas chromatograph equipped with a split injector and a flame ionization detector (Hewlett-Packard Co., Palo Alto, CA). The column used was a 15 m x 0.32 mm (i.d.), 0.25 µm DB-5. The temperature programme used was: initial temperature was 170^{0}C (1 min), 5^{0}C/min to 230^{0}C, 20^{0}C/min to 290^{0}C where the temperature was kept for 10 min. The peaks were integrated using a Hewlett-Packard 3396A Integrator. The amount of ethyl palmitate, ethyl stearate, ethyl oleate and ethyl linoleate was calculated from the ratio between the ethyl ester peak and the peak of the internal standard (nonadecanoic acid ethyl ester), using a standard curve for each ethyl ester.

Results

Formation of FAEEs in rat and human liver microsomes

Biochemical characterization of AEAT activity

As mentioned above, two enzymatic activities are involved in the formation of FAEEs in vitro, which were biochemically characterized using isolated rat and human liver microsomes. We first aimed at optimizing the method for measuring AEAT activity. Parameters such as varying concentrations of ethanol and [1-14C]palmitoyl-CoA (the substrates), amount of microsomal protein, albumin concentration, and changing the incubation time were determined. The highest AEAT activity was found with 100 μM palmitoyl-CoA, and at concentrations higher than 100 μM the AEAT activity was slightly inhibited (Figure 1). The optimal concentration of ethanol was between 0.5 and 1.25 M (not shown). Above 1.25 M ethanol, the AEAT activity was severely decreased, probably interfering with membrane structures and substrate solubility. The concentration of ethanol chosen for the AEAT assay was 0.86 M. Based on these results, a standard AEAT assay was designed (described in Methods) which was used throughout unless otherwise indicated.

A striking finding was that measurement of maximal AEAT activity requires addition of BNPP (which is a common serine esterase inhibitor) into the incubation mixture. In the presence of 250 μM BNPP, AEAT activity was increased about six-fold using rat liver microsomes, and two-fold when using human liver microsomes, respectively (Figure 2). This apparent stimulation of AEAT activity is due to inhibition of microsomal acyl-CoA hydrolase activity which, in the absence of BNPP, competes with AEAT for the same substrate (palmitoyl-CoA). It has previously been shown that the major microsomal acyl-CoA hydrolase activity in rat liver is due to carboxylesterase ES-4, which is inhibited by BNPP and p-HMB (Berge, 1979; Mentlein, et al., 1984; Alexson, et al., 1993). Thus, inhibition of acyl-CoA hydrolase activity by BNPP allows measurement of the maximal capacity of AEAT. Another potent microsomal acyl-CoA-hydrolase inhibitor, p-HMB (which is a cysteine-reacting agent) exerted a similar apparent stimulatory effect on AEAT activity in rat liver microsomes (Figure 2). However, AEAT activity was inhibited by p-HMB in human liver microsomes, suggesting that the AEAT activity is due to different enzyme(s) in human and rat liver microsomes.
AEAT activity was significantly higher in isolated human liver microsomes than in rat liver microsomes when measured in the absence of BNPP (16.5 and 1.7 nmol/min x mg protein, respectively). When BNPP was included in the incubations the AEAT activity was 32 nmol/min x mg protein in human liver microsomes and about 10 nmol/min x mg protein in rat liver microsomes (Table 1). The weaker stimulatory effect of BNPP on AEAT activity in human liver microsome could possibly be explained by lower acyl-CoA hydrolase activity. We therefore

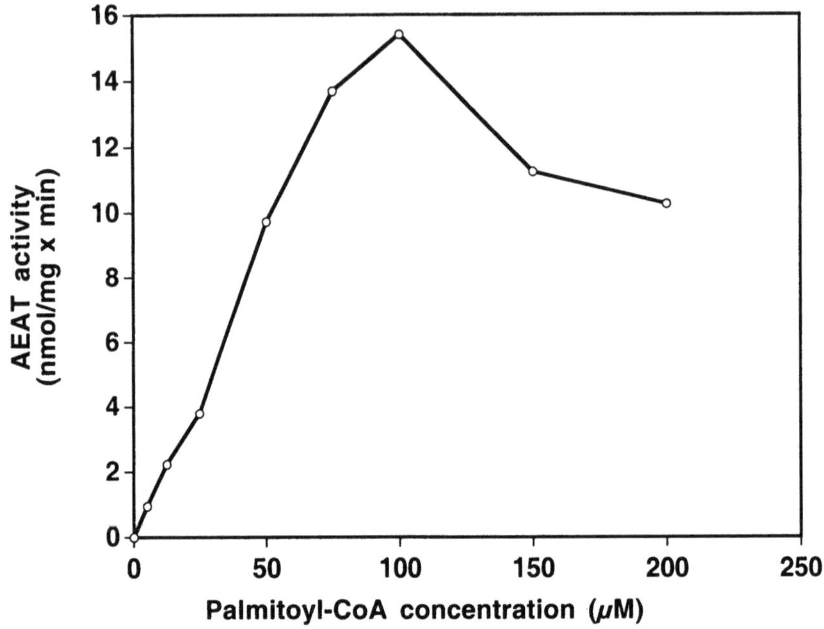

Figure 1 Effect of varying substrate concentration on AEAT activity. AEAT activity was determined as described in Methods, using rat liver microsomes incubated with [14C]palmitoyl-CoA at the concentrations indicated. BNPP (250 μM) was included in the incubations in order to measure maximal activity.

performed Western blot analysis on human liver microsomes, using monospecific peptide antibodies directed against rat ES-4, which showed no reactivity in human liver microsomes, indicating that ES-4 is not expressed in humans.

Effects of an ACAT inhibitor on AEAT activity

DL-Melinamide is a potent acyl-CoA; cholesterol *O*-acyltransferase (ACAT) inhibitor. Incubation of rat liver microsomes with DL-melinamide resulted in a strong inhibition of AEAT activity. The IC50 value for AEAT inhibition was 2.5 μM, being about the same as for inhibition of ACAT (Diczfalusy, et al., 1999). However, AEAT activity i human liver microsomes was not inhibited by DL-melinamide, again suggesting possible differences in the rat and human AEAT proteins.

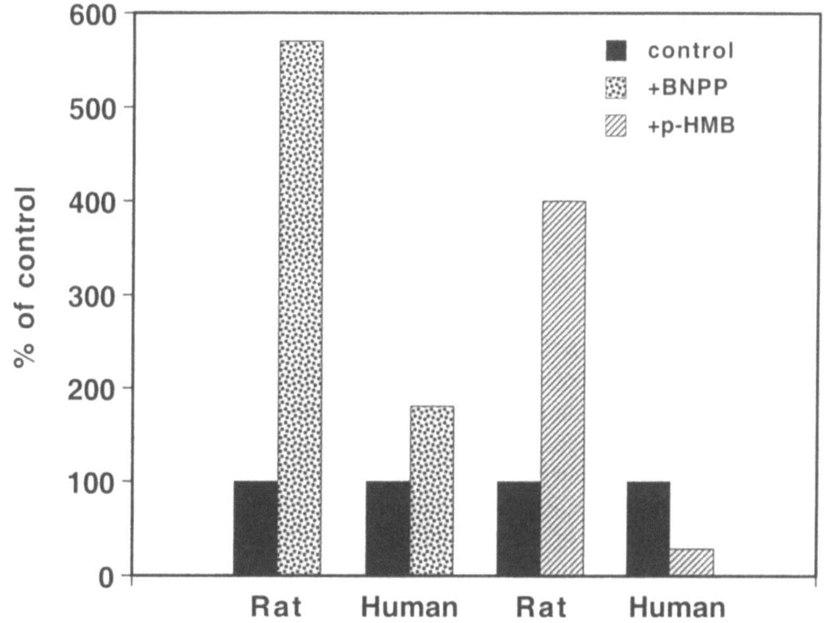

Figure 2 Effect of BNPP and p-HMB on AEAT activity in rat and human liver microsomes. AEAT activity was measured as described in Methods. Microsomes were preincubated for 15 minutes with the serine esterase inhibitor BNPP or the cysteine targeting reagent p-HMB. Substrates (100 μM [1-14C]palmitoyl-CoA and 0.86 M ethanol) were then added and the samples were incubated for another 15 minutes. The effects are shown as % of control incubations performed in the absence of BNPP and p-HMB.

	AEAT	**FAEE synthase**	**FAEE hydrolase**
Rat liver microsomes	1.7 nmol/min x mg protein	1.7 nmol/min x mg protein	97 nmol/min x mg protein
Human liver Microsomes	16.5 nmol/min x mg protein	1.7 nmol/min x mg protein	40.1 nmol/min x mg protein

Diczfalusy M. A., Björkhem I., Einarsson C. and Alexson, S. E. H. Formation of fatty acid ethyl esters in rat liver microsomes. Evidence for a key role of acyl-CoA: ethanol *O*-acyltransferase. *Eur. J. Biochem.* **259**, 404-411.

Table 1 Fatty acid ethyl ester synthesizing and hydrolyzing activities in rat and human liver microsomes. AEAT and FAEE synthase activities were determinded in isolated microsomes as described in Methods. The activities are given as means of four to seven preparaions, each measured in duplicate from (Diczfalusy, et al., 1999) and Diczfalusy et al., submitted for publication.

FAEE synthase activity

The FAEE synthase activity in isolated rat liver microsomes was found to be in the same range as the AEAT activity when measured in the absence of BNPP (1.7 nmol/min x mg microsomal protein). FAEE synthase activity in human liver microsomes was about 3 nmol/min x mg microsomal protein. The synthesis of ethyl palmitate by FAEE synthase was inhibited in the presence of 250 μM BNPP. The inhibition by BNPP suggests that FAEE synthase contains an active site serine involved in the catalytic action of the protein, and may be identical to one of the microsomal carboxylesterases as suggested by others (Tsujita and Okuda, 1992). However, we have purified two of the rat liver microsomal carboxylesterases, carboxylesterase ES-4 and ES-10, which were found to possess very low (if any) FAEE synthase activity [for details see (Diczfalusy, et al., 1999)]. FAEE synthase activity was not affected by p-HMB.

Hydrolysis of fatty acid ethyl esters

Rat liver microsomes contain several carboxylesterases which are able to hydrolyze a wide range of different lipid esters (Mentlein, et al., 1984). Therefore we examined the rate of hydrolysis of ethyl palmitate in human and rat liver microsomes. Our results showed that the hydrolysis of ethyl palmitate was 97 nmol/min x mg protein in rat liver microsomes and 40 nmol/min x mg protein in human liver microsomes. We further investigated the effect of BNPP and p-HMB on the FAEE hydrolyzing activity. BNPP completely inhibited the hydrolysis but p-HMB had no effect on the hydrolysis in human liver microsomes, while it completely inhibited the hydrolysis of FAEEs in rat liver microsomes (tested at 40 μM concentration). These results show that human liver microsomes have a much higher capacatity to synthesize ethyl esters than rat liver microsomes, and that the hydrolyzing activity of formed ethyl esters is lower in human liver microsomes. The combined effects of these two enzyme activities may facilitate formation and accumulation of FAEEs in human liver. We therefore investigated the activities of FAEE-synthesizing and hydrolyzing activities in homogenates of various human tissues.

FAEE-synthesizing and hydrolyzing activities in human organs

Total tissue homogenates were prepared from several human tissues and AEAT, FAEE-synthase and FAEE hydrolase activities were measured (Diczfalusy et al., submitted for publication). These activities were measured in intestine, liver, heart and pancreas (Figure 3A). AEAT activity was higher than FAEE synthase activity in all tissues tested. The AEAT activity was clearly higher in liver (being about 400 nmol/min x g tissue) than in all other tissues, and found to be about 5-fold higher than FAEE synthase activity. Also intestine contained high AEAT activity (about 120 nmol/min x g tissue), while FAEE synthase activity was near the level of detection. In contrast, AEAT and FAEE synthase activities were similar in pancreas. Liver and pancreas contained the clearly highest FAEE hydrolyzing activities (being about 1100 nmol/min x g tissue in both organs), while the hydrolyzing activities were low in intestine and heart (Figure 3B). These data suggest that liver and intestine may be the primary sites for FAEE synthesis, and the very low FAEE hydrolyzing activity in intestine indicate that this organ may produce FAEEs that could potentially be secreted into the blood. Since FAEEs have been reported to appear in blood after ethanol intake, we also measured FAEE synthesizing and hydrolyzing activities in serum samples from humans and rats (Diczfalusy et al., submitted for publication). Human and rat serum was found to have negligible AEAT and FAEE synthase activities. Human serum also contained very low FAEE hydrolase activity, in contrast, rat serum contained very high FAEE hydrolyzing activity. Similar to human sera, AEAT and FAEE synthase activities were negligible in sera from rats. Taken together these data indicate that FAEEs synthesized in various human organs may be secreted to blood, where the FAEE hydrolyzing activity is low, which could account for the observed accumulation of FAEEs in humans during alcohol intake.

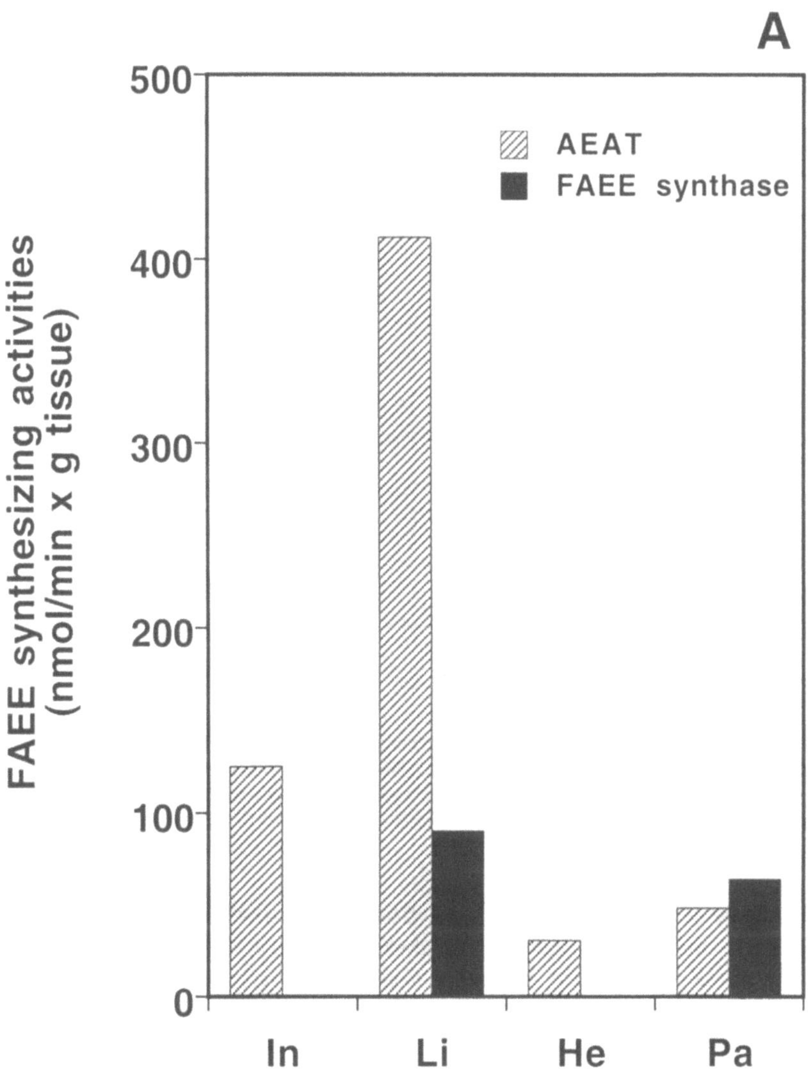

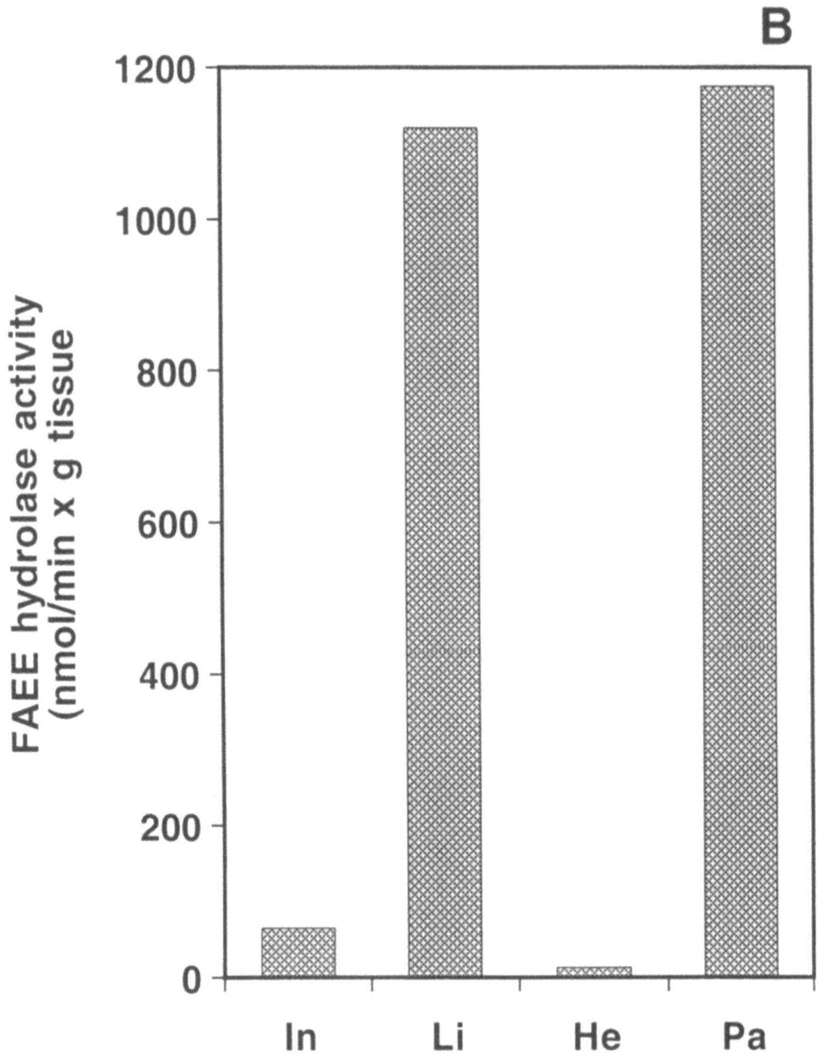

Figure 3 FAEE synthesizing and hydrolyzing activities in human tissue homogenates. Total homogenates were prepared from intestine (In), liver (Li), heart (He) and pancreas (Pa) and incubated (in the absence of BNPP) for AEAT and FAEE synthase activities (A) and FAEE hydrolyzing (B) activities. Note that the FAEE synthase activity was to low in intestine and heart to show up in the histogram.

Appearance of FAEEs in blood during ethanol intake

In order to study the appearence and disappearence of FAEEs in blood during alcohol intake, one healthy volunteer (fasted overnight) ingested 160 ml 40% alcohol as 4 aliquots which were administered during 45 minutes. Blood samples were collected and analyzed for FAEEs and blood ethanol. Blood ethanol leveles were rapidly elevated and reached a peak value of nearly 20 mM at 60 minutes (Figures 4).

The blood ethanol level then rapidly decreased and no ethanol could be detected at 24 hours. Blood FAEEs were separated and quantitated using GC. Also FAEEs increased rapidly and reached a peak at 60 - 90 minutes, whereafter the FAEEs declined (Figure 4b). Strikingly, the FAEEs increased again after 190 minutes, apparently coinciding with the meal at 240 minutes. The second peak of FAEEs occurred at 300 minutes after which the levels slowly decreased. However, still at 24 hours there were detectable levels of FAEEs, in contrast to blood ethanol which was not detectable at this timepoint

Using GC, the various fatty acid species of FAEEs could be separated and quantitated. The predominant fatty acids were found to be oleate, stearate and palmitate, while linoleate levels were lower. Strikingly, FAEEs of the saturated fatty acids (stearate and palmitate) remained elevated even at 24 hours, while FAEEs containing unsaturated fatty acids disappeared faster and could not be detected at this timepoint.

Figures 4 Apperance of FAEEs in blood during ethanol intake

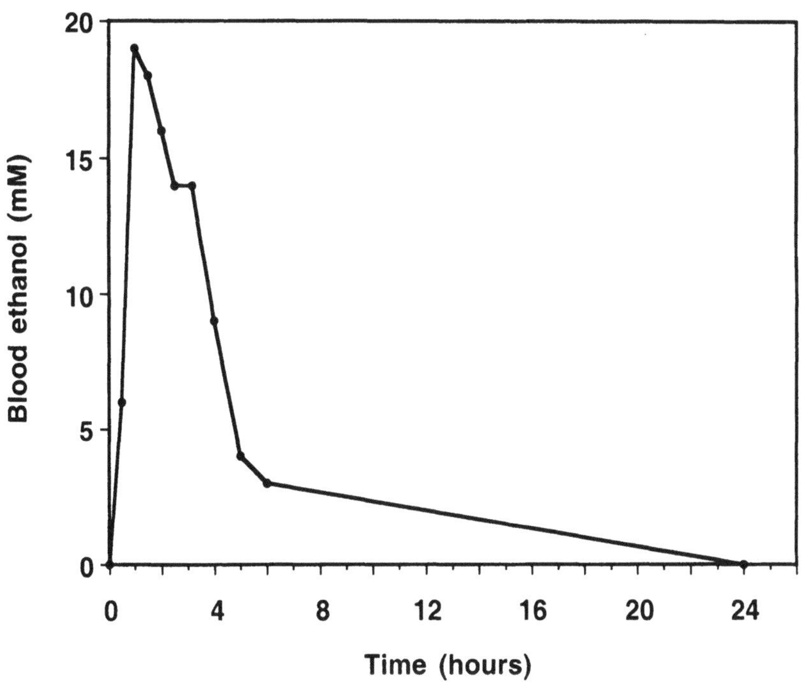

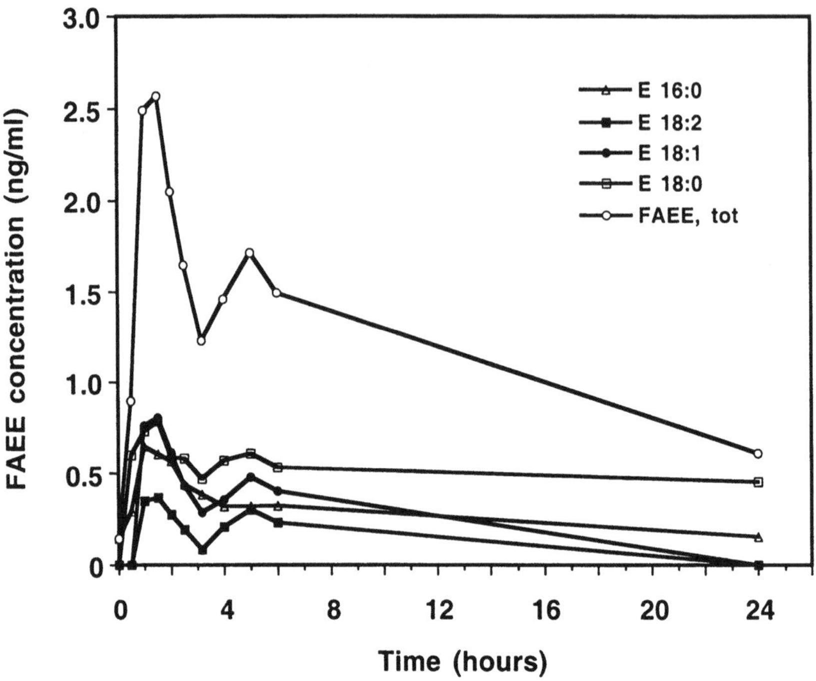

Discussion

FAEEs have been shown to accumulate in blood during alcohol intake (Doyle, et al., 1994; Doyle, et al., 1996; Soderberg, et al., 1999). Still the site of synthesis and the enzymes involved in esterifcation of fatty acids to ethanol in vivo are unknown. Most previous studies have focused on FAEE synthase and only limited information is available about FAEE synthesis via AEAT. FAEE synthases have been purified from various tissues and organisms and in most cases been identified as carboxylesterases (Tsujita and Okuda, 1992; Bora, et al., 1996; Kaphalia, et al., 1997). However, our results strongly suggest that AEAT is likely to be the most important activity in both rat and human, based on the general observation that in all comparisons AEAT activity is higher than FAEE synthase activity. Also, cultured HepG2 cells have been shown to synthesize FAEEs from ethanol added to the culture medium, mainly via AEAT (Kabakibi, et al., 1998). Still conclusive evidence for the formation of FAEEs by AEAT in vivo is lacking, but there are indirect data supporting that AEAT is most important. Under normal nutritional conditions, fatty acids liberated from triacylglycerols are rapidly converted to acyl-CoAs which are reesterified with other lipid alcohols. Accordingly, the concentration of acyl-CoAs within the cell can be expected to be much higher than the concentration of free fatty acids. Studies on the formation of dicarboxylic acids, which are exclusively formed from free fatty acids by microsomal ω-hydroxylation, demonstrated that very little of these acids are formed under normal conditions. In contrast, during fasting and diabetes, the synthesis of dicarboxylic fatty acids is markedly increased, apparently due to the increased levels of non-esterified fatty acids under ketotic conditions (Bjorkhem, 1976; Wada, et al., 1971). It is therefore possible that synthesis of FAEEs by FAEE synthase may become more important under conditions when free fatty acids are increased, e.g. during fasting.

From measurements of FAEE synthase and AEAT activities in various human organs, it appears that intestine may be an important site of synthesis and possible secretion to blood. This is supported by the findings of rather high AEAT activity in intestinal mucosa, and a strikingly low FAEE hydrolase activity. Considering the importance of the intestinal mucosa in esterification of fatty acids into complex lipids (triacylglycerol, phospholipids and cholesteryl esters) it is plausible that fatty acids may also to a large extent be esterified to ethanol as a side-reaction. As the esterified lipids produced in the intestine are secreted to the circulation for transport to peripheral tissues, this route of delivery may also apply to FAEEs. The low FAEE hydrolyzing activity in serum could allow for accumulation of FAEEs in blood, as observed in humans during alcohol intake.

The possible role of FAEEs as mediators of organ injury is still unclear. Normally only low levels of FAEEs can be detected in various human organs, with the exception of adipose tissue which contain rather high levels also in "social drinkers" (Laposata and Lange, 1986). Strongly elevated FAEE levels can be detected in a number of organs with low, or no, capacity to oxidize ethanol. Although these organs (e.g. heart) also appear to have low capacities to synthesize FAEEs, low hydrolyzing activities may allow accumulation of FAEEs during acute ethanol intake. In vitro data show that FAEEs may have detrimental effects on cell function, lysosome fragility in pancreas and that FAEEs can uncouple mitochondria (Lange and Sobel, 1983; Szczypiorkowski, et al., 1995; Haber, et al., 1993). Still, however, no good experimental model is available to test this hypothesis. One possibility would be to use the ACAT inhibitor DL-melinamide, which is a potent inhibitor also of rat liver microsomal AEAT in vitro. If this inhibitor is active also in vivo in rats, its effect on synthesis of FAEEs during alcohol intake, and possible protection against organ injury could be studied.

Several biological markers of alcohol intake have been identified and studied such as gamma glutamyl transferase, mean corpuscular volume, ALAT and carbohydrate deficient transferrin. The sensitivity and specificity of these tests to detect ethanol ingestion have however been unsatisfactory. There is a need for tests that are specific for ethanol intake which are not affected by physiological or pharmacological factors and which are sensitive enough to detect excess alcohol consumption. Most markers currently used are unlikely to be useful in individuals infrequently ingesting small amounts of alcohol. However, these markers can be used as long-term markers to detect high ethanol intake during a long period of time. In contrast, FAEEs can be detected after a single episode of modest alcohol intake. In accordance with previous results by Laposatas group (Doyle, et al., 1996; Doyle, et al., 1994), our data suggest that FAEE levels remain elevated in blood for some time after blood ethanol levels are undetectable. Although our present data does not allow a firm conclusion, they indicate that elevated levels of FAEEs may be detected up to about 10 hours after ethanol have disappeared from the blood. Thus, FAEEs may be used as a short term marker for ethanol intake.

Acknowledgements

We are grateful to Ms. Inger Moberg for excellent help with analysis of fatty acid ethyl esters. This work was supported by the Swedish Medical Research Council, the Swedish Natural Science Research Council, the Swedish Research Council for Engineering Sciences and Svenska Sällskapet for Medicinsk Forskning.

References

Alexson S. E. H., Mentlein R., Wernstedt C. and Hellman U. 1993 Isolation and characterization of microsomal acyl-CoA thioesterase: A member of the rat liver microsomal carboxylesterase multigene family. Eur. J. Biochem. 214, 719-727.

Berge R. K. 1979 Purification and characterization of a long-chain acyl-CoA hydrolase from rat liver microsomes. Biochim. Biophys. Acta 574, 321-333.

Björkhem I. 1976 On the mechanism of regulation of ω-oxidation of fatty acids. J. Biol. Chem. 251, 5259-5266.

Bora P. S., Guruge D. G., Miller D. D., Chaitman B. R. and Ruyle M. S. 1996 Purification and characterization of human heart fatty acid ethyl ester synthase/carboxylesterase. J. Mol. Cell Cardiol. 28, 2027-2032.

Bora P. S., Spilburg C. A. and Lange L. G. 1989 Metabolism of ethanol and carcinogens by glutathione transferases. Prot. Natl. Acad. Sci. USA 86, 4470-4473.

Bradford M. M. 1976 A rapid and sensitive method for the quantitation of microgram quantities of protein utilizing the principle of protein/dye binding. Anal. Biochem. 72, 248-254.

Chang W., Waltenbaugh C. and Borensztajn J. 1997 Fatty acid ethyl ester synthesis by isolated perfused rat heart. Metabolism 46, 926-929.

Dan L. and Laposata M. 1997 Ethyl palmitate and ethyl oleate are the predominant fatty acid ethyl esters in the blood after ethanol ingestion and their synthesis is differentially influenced by the extracellular concentrations of their corresponding fatty acids. Alcohol. Clin. Exp. Res. 21; 2, 286-292.

Diczfalusy M. A., Björkhem I., Einarsson C. and Alexson S. E. H. 1999 Formation of fatty acid ethyl esters in rat liver microsomes. Evidence for a key role of acyl-CoA : ethanol O-acyltransferase. Eur. J. Biochem. 259, 404-411.

Doyle K. M., Bird D. A., Al-Salihi S., Hallaq J., Cluette-Brown J. E., Goss K. A. and Laposata M. 1994 Fatty acid ethyl esters are present in human serum after ethanol ingestion. J. Lipid Res. 35, 428-437.

Doyle K. M., Cluette-Brown J. E., Dube D. M., Bernhard T. G., Morse C. R. and Laposata M. 1996 Fatty acid ethyl esters in the blood as markers for ethanol intake. J.A.M.A. 276, 1152-1156.

Einarsson K., Benthin L., Ewerth S., Hellers G., Stahlberg D. and Angelin B. 1989 Studies on acyl-coenzyme A:cholesterol acyltransferase activity in human liver microsomes. J. Lipid Res. 30, 739-746.

Haber P. S., Wilson J. S., Apte M. V. and Pirola R. C. 1993 Fatty acid ethyl esters increase rat pancreatic lysosomal fragility. J. Lab. Clin. Med. 121, 759-764.

Kabakibi A., Morse C. R. and Laposata M. 1998 Fatty acid ethyl esters and HepG2 cells: intracellular synthesis and release from the cells. J. Lipid Res. 39, 1568-1582.

Kaphalia B. S., Fritz R. R. and Ansari G. A. S. 1997 Purification and characterization of rat liver microsomal fatty acid ethyl and 2-chloroethyl ester synthase and their relationship with carboxylesterase (pI 6.1). Chem. Res. Toxicol. 10, 211-218.

Lange L. G. and Sobel B. 1983 Mitochondrial dysfunction induced by fatty acid ethyl esters, myocardial metabolites of ethanol. J. Clin. Invest. 72, 724-731.

Laposata E. A. and Lange L. G. 1986 Presence of nonoxidative ethanol metabolism in human organs commonly damaged by ethanol abuse. Science 231, 497-499.

Lieber C. S. 1985 Alcohol and the liver: metabolism of ethanol, metabolic effects and pathogenesis of injury. Acta Med. Scand. Suppl. 703, 11-55.

Mentlein R., Suttorp M. and Heymann E. 1984 Specificity of purified monoacylglycerol lipase, palmitoyl-CoA hydrolase, palmitoyl-carnitine hydrolase, and nonspecific carboxylesterase from rat liver microsomes. Arch. Biochem. Biophys. 228, 230-246.

Polokoff M. A. and Bell R. M. 1978 Limited palmitoyl-CoA penetration into microsomal vesicles as evidenced by a high latent ethanol acyltransferase activity. J. Biol. Chem. 253, 7173-7178.

Riley D. J. S., Kyger E. M., Spilburg C. A. and Lange L. G. 1990 Pancreatic cholesterol esterases. 2. Purification and characterization of human pancreatic fatty acid ethyl ester synthase. Biochemistry 29, 3848-3852.

Soderberg B. L., Sicinska E. T., Blodget E., Cluette-Brown J. E., Suter P. M., Schuppisser T., Vetter W. and Laposata M. 1999 Preanalytical variables affecting the quantification of fatty acid ethyl esters in plasma and serum samples. Clin. Chem. 45, 2183-2190.

Szczypiorkowski Z. M., Dickersin G. R. and Laposata M. 1995 Fatty acid ethyl esters decrease human hopatoblastoma cell proliferation and protein synthesis. Gastroenterology 108, 515-522.

Tsujita T. and Okuda H. 1992 Fatty acid ethyl ester synthase in rat adipose tissue and its relationship to carboxylesterase. J. Biol. Chem. 267, 23489-23494.

Tsujita T. and Okuda H. 1994 The synthesis of fatty acid ethyl ester by carboxylester lipase. Eur. J. Biochem. 224, 57-62.

Wada F., Usami M., Goto M. and Hayashi T. 1971 Studies on the physiological significance of fatty acid ω-oxidation. J. Biochem. 70, 1065-1067.

Methanol and congeners as markers of alcohol use and abuse

Thomas Gilg

Institut für Rechtsmedizin
Ludwig Maximilans Universität München
Frauenlobstrasse 7 a
80337 München

Phone: +49-89-5160 5111
FAX: +49-89-5160 5144
Email: gilg@rechts.med.uni-muenchen.de

Abstract

Congener analysis and especially methanol contribute to evaluate and differentiate a declared consumption of various alcoholic beverages, e.g. to judge post offence drinking claims. Methanol with serum (or urinary) levels exceeding 10 mg /l cannot be achieved by short time drinking, except with fruit brandy (which can be identified by concomitantly elevated levels of butanol - 2 and MEK (methyl ethyl ketone, as its metabolic product). Numerous results and experiences indicate that methanol, as well as acetone > 7 mg / l and isopropanol > 2 mg / l resp. acetone + isopropanol > 9 mg / l, are markers for recent heavy drinking resp. long periods of alcoholization. At least they indicate alcohol abuse in blood or urine samples taken in alcoholized states or in earlier phases (hours) after drinking. The biological turnover (half time Apr. 2, 4 hours in methanol) has to be considered, which – as generally in marker studies – may affect the outcome of studies with respect to sensitivity. Its main use is more the detection of heavy prolonged drinking as in traffic and social medicine and in intensive care units to recognize possible withdrawals than as a relapse marker. It fits in the time screen of other markers as a short time marker. Methanol metabolism presents interesting aspects in view of the development of addiction and dependency (influence on the C1 metabolism) as well as on hangover and withdrawal.

Introduction

Alcoholic beverages contain numerous other substances, but in considerably lower concentrations than ethanol. These are e.g. higher alcohols, esters, flavonoides, amines and others, usually addressed as fusel oils or congeners (Bonte and Hey, 1983, Gilg, 1999, Greenberg, 1970, Nykänen and Suolomainen, 1983a ,b). They are not only characteristic for types of beverages, aroma, flavour and taste, but also a significant factor for tolerability and hangover. According to reports and own experiences, hangover symptoms are more severe after consumption of congener rich beverages than after nearly pure vodka (Bonte, 1987, Gilg, 1992, Gilg, 1993, Gilg et al., 1995)
After preliminary investigations by Machata (Machata and Prokop, 1971) it was mainly German institutes of forensic medicine, with Bonte as a pioneer, who performed basic research on congeners since 1978 (Barz, 1993, Bilzer et al., 1990, Bonte, 1987, Gilg, 1986, Gilg, 1995, Gilg et al., 1995, Gilg, 1999, Grüner and Bilzer, 1985 Iffland et al., 1984, Iffland et al., 1989, Iffland and Staak, 1990, Iffland 1993, Iffland et al., 1994). The initial question from a practical view was, whether methods could be established to evaluate the so called "hip flask" drinking - which means an alcohol consumption after an accident resp. after drunken driving, that may be discharging of an accused DUI or DWI (driving under the influence resp. while intoxicated). According to established pharmacological and pharmacokinetic criteria, the congeners as listed below were found to be of practical value for evaluation and are part of routine diagnosis and evaluation in many German institutes of forensic medicine since years. As an example, in our institute we have to deal with 350 files annually concerning congeners and methanol since more than 15 years.
Figure 1 shows characteristic profiles of those congeners in classes of alcoholic beverages.

Besides congener rich beverages like fruit brandy there are nearly congener free drinks like vodka, grain or also liqueurs (Bonte, 1987). Main problem is, that due to fermentation principles and substrates there are practically no indicative congeners for single drinks or characteristic classes of beverages, except butanol - 2, which is found nearly only in fruit brandy. Therefore an evaluation is mostly based on quantitative differences in contents and resulting blood levels, e.g. predominantly propanol - 1 in / after beer - or isobutanol in / after wine resp. more concentrated in brandy due to destillation.
After bolus respectively short time consumption of either beer, white wine, brandy, fruit brandy or vodka, typical concentrations in serum are found (Figure 2). The subjects reached blood alcohol concentrations (BAC) of approximately 1 to 1, 3 ‰. In more or less ideal situations, e.g., if somebody claims a consumption of relevant amounts of fruit brandy after an accident, we definitely have to expect equivalent levels in serum or blood. In case we find a typical „bavarian beer spectrum“ like on top of figure 2 and no equivalent values of methanol, propanol - 1, butanol - 2 and methyl-ethyl-ketone (MEK), the statement has to be rejected.

Different drinking habits have to be evaluated by calculating presumed blood levels and by comparison with experiences and results of drinking experiments.

Typical contents of congeners in different classes of alcoholic beverages (mod. Acc. to BONTE 1987)

Beverage	MeOH	Prop-1	But-2	Isobut	2-M-B-1	3-M-B-1
Beer	**7 ± 3**	13 ± 3	0	13 ± 4	13 ± 3	52 ± 12
Wheat beer	**4 - 22**	10 - 30	0	9 - 85	8 - 28	34 - 84
White wine	**29 ± 16**	31 ± 8	0	56 ± 18	27 ± 6	112 ± 25
Red wine	**104 ± 30**	30 ± 7	0 - 1	47 ± 15	33 ± 6	137 ± 26
Champagne	**16 ± 8**	31 ± 5	0	53 ± 15	30 ± 7	126 ± 28
Brandy	**272 ± 76**	130 ± 22	1 - 18	252 ± 38	77 - 186	482 - 961
Cognac	**273 ± 97**	184 ± 23	0 - 6	385 ± 56	125 ± 33	764 ± 86
Whisky (Scotch)	**112 ± 19**	171 ± 29	0	263 ± 36	59 ± 12	239 ± 44
Whiskey (US)	**196 - 328**	50 - 193	0	388 ± 99	271 ± 53	1059 ±
Fruit brandy	**562 - 1642**	82 - 267	**41 - 430**	12 - 336	12 - 202	58 - 1073
Pear brandy	**3783 ± 983**	**1382 ± 686**	**609 ± 479**	210 ± 71	65 ± 21	307 ± 131
Rye	**4 - 95**	0 - 6	0	0 - 1	0 - 10	0 - 16
Vodka	**1 - (170)**	0 (-16)	0	0	0	0

Figure 1 Contents of congeners in classes of alcoholic beverages in mg/l., MeOH = Methanol, Prop-1 = propanol-1, But-2 = Butanol-2 (secondary butanol), Isobut = Isobutanol, 2-M-B-1 = 2-Methyl-Butanol-1, 3-M-B-1 = 3-Methyl-Butanol-1

The corresponding pharmacokinetic criteria are too complex to be listed here (comp. Bilzer et al., 1990, Bonte, 1987 and reports mainly in Blutalkohol) - except referring to methanol, which is of special interest and will be discussed in detail as follows.

The basis of evaluation is a sensitive and specific analysis like Head Space Gaschromatography, which is basically used. Normal Head Space Gaschromatography (GC) is routinely used and optimized for the determination of blood alcohol resp. ethanol, with concentrations being more than a thousand times higher than in congeners. Routine blood alcohol analysis may detect congeners including methanol from 10 mg / l on, - as well as isopropanol, acetone and other volatile substances in relevant concentrations. These screening results

have to be assured by a more specific and sensitive, special GC - method like congener analysis, identifying and quantifying numerous volatile substances including methanol, ethanol, acetaldehyde and others with detection limits as low as 0, 02 mg / l resp. 0, 2 mg / l for methanol (details in Gilg, 1992, Gilg et al., 1995).

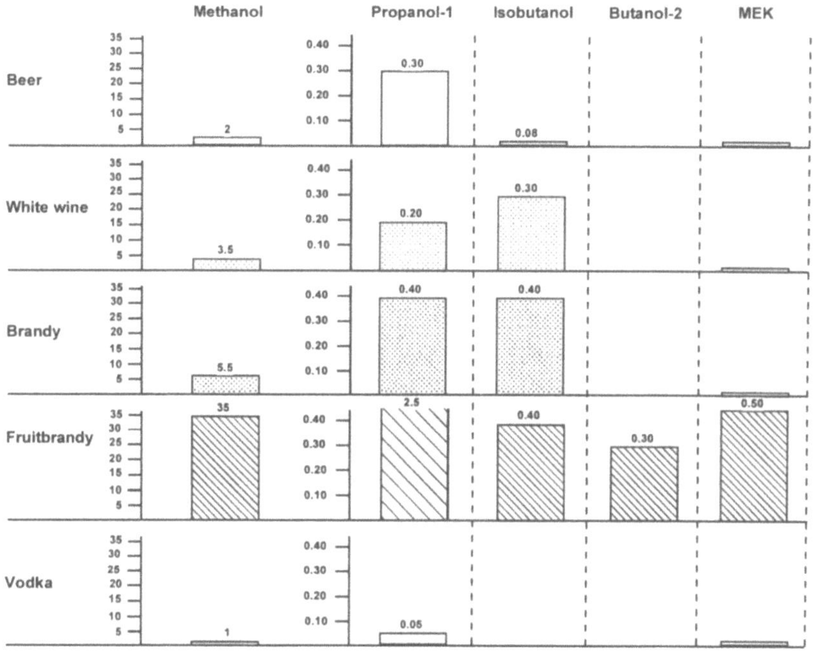

Figure 2 Diagram of typical concentrations of congeners in serum after bolus intake (1-1,5 hours) of either beer, white or red wine, fruit brandy or vodka, with BAC of appr. 1-1,3 ‰

Acetaldehyde as the first elimination product is not suitable to give information on the phase or extent of ethanol metabolism, even if an enzymatic build up in vitro is blocked by special sample taking and preparation, which is a prerequisite (DiPadova et al., 1984, Eriksson, 1980, Eriksson, 1983)). Levels found in congener analysis are low and uncharacteristic, they show no correlation with BAC, but are elevated in hemolized samples (Fischer and Kampmann, 1982, Gilg, 1995, Gilg et al., 1995). Only in cases with an inefficient type of aldehydedehydrogenase resp. ALDH, as in 10 - 20 % of asians, characteristically elevated levels can be found after alcohol consumption (Inoue et al., 1984), as well as after intake of antabus - like drugs (Fischer and Kampmann, 1982).
Otherwise acetaldehyde has been incriminated as a reason for hangover, which still may be an interesting hypothesis considering increased ethanol elimination in alcoholics with possibly elevated levels of acetaldehyde resp. unknown intra cellular effects, acetaldehyde adducts or a formation of TIQ (tetrahydroisoquinolines), which also may derive from formaldehyde as the metabolic product in methanol metabolism (Bonte et al., 1988, Bonte et al., 1991, Gilg, 1995, Gilg et

al., 1995, Musshoff et al., 1995). In comparison methanol is highly resistent to in-vitro and post-mortem changes (Meyer at al., 1994), even when signs of putrefaction with a build up of other congeners are present (Bonte and Hey, 1983). Pure theoretical considerations like from Stöhlmacher (1996) cannot underline an indirect or even direct formation ot methanol from ethanol.
Acetate as the metabolic product of acetaldehyde is also proposed as alcohol marker (Korri et al., 1985, Lands, 1991), but not investigated as detailed as others, tampered also by analytical problems outside routines.

In absence of ethanol congeners are eliminated so fast, that they are nearly not detectable in blood (Bonte, 1987). The presence of relevant BAC causes an incomplete inhibition of metabolism, so congeners become detectable. Methanol metabolism plays a special role because of its complete inhibition by ethanol. It is a well known fact from the treatment of methanol intoxications, that ethanol of at least 0, 2 to 0, 5 ‰, better 1 ‰, leads to a complete competitive inhibition of the ADH (alcoholdehydrogenase) - related, enzymatic degradation of methanol. This reduces the metabolic production of the main toxic metabolite, which - by the way - is strongly supposed not to be formaldehyde, but formic acid. Expectations were realistic, that the same effect should happen in methanol concentrations much lower than toxic levels (which usually exceed 500 mg/l methanol in blood). First investigations on human methanol metabolism with non toxic levels began already in the early seventies by Majchrowicz and Magrinat (Magrinat, 1973, Majchrowicz and Mendelson, 1970, Majchrowicz and Sutherland, 1971, Majchrowicz and Mendelson, 1971, Majchrowicz and Steinglass, 1973, Machrowicz, 1975) as well as Pieper and Skeen (1973) in chimpanzees (in general species differences esp. in studies on methanol metabolism in rats have to be considered, Rietbrock, 1969, Roe, 1982). Elevated methanol levels were detected in those studies and connections with withdrawal symptoms were discussed.
Further research since 1982 was underwent by Bilzer et al.(1991), Bonte and Barz (Barz, 1993, Bonte, 1987, Bonte et al, 1988, Bonte, 1991), Gilg (Gilg, 1986, Gilg et al., 1987, Gilg et al., 1987, Gilg et al, 1989, Gilg, 1992, Gilg, 1995, Gilg et al., 1995, Gilg, 1999), Grüner (Grüner and Bilzer, 1982, Grüner and Bilzer, 1985, Grüner et al., 1993), Haffner (Haffner et al., 1993, 1996, 1997a,b,c, 1998), Iffland (Iffland et al., 1984, 1989, 1994, Iffland and Staak, 1990, Iffland, 1993), Jones (Jones, 1983, Jones et al., 1987, Jones, 1987, Jones and Löwinger, 1988, Jones et al., 1989, Jones and Sternebring, 1992, Jones and Helander, 1998), Musshoff et al. (1995), Roine et al. (1989), Sprung (Sprung et al., 1988, Sprung and Bonte, 1988) and Tsokos et al. (1996) gave a clearer picture of the practical importance and relevance of methanol (and besides isopropanol/acetone). Outside Europe and especially Germany research on methanol to this respect is underreported and – estimated, there are only occasional reports (Lindinger et al., 1997, Wargotz and Werner, 1987), or letters (Collins, 1990).

The basic results are presented exemplarily in the following.
A short time resp. bolus consumption of beer, white or red wine leads to only moderate methanol levels well below 10 mg /l (Figure 3). Only methanol rich beverages like fruit brandy may lead to levels > 10 mg/l (comp. Figure 2 and Figure 7).

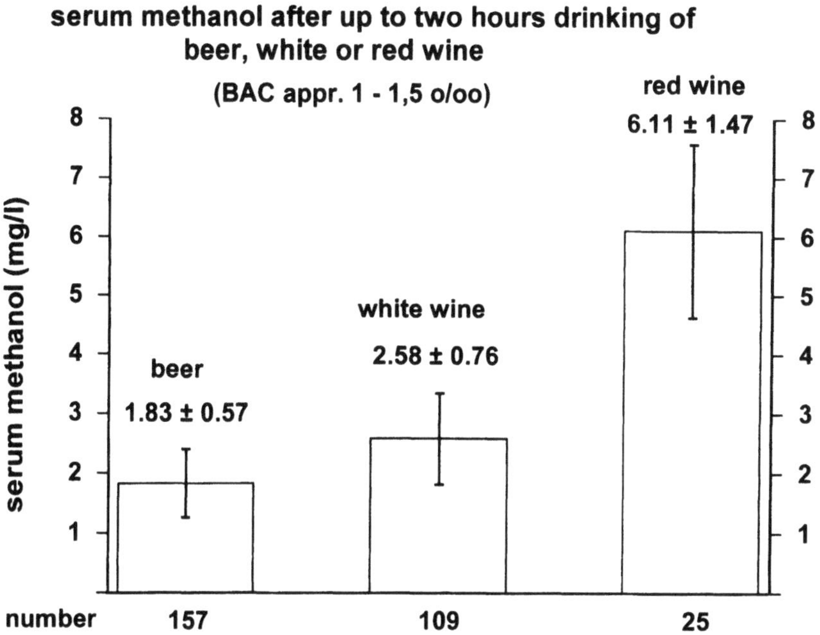

Figure 3 Serum methanol after bolus consumption of beer, white or red wine with levels well below 10 mg/l

On the other hand there is a strong coincidence between higher BAC and elevated methanol in drunken drivers even without consumption of fruit brandies (Gilg, 1992, Gilg, 1995, Gilg et al., 1995, Grüner and Bilzer, 1982, 1995, Iffland et al., 1984, Iffland and Staak, 1990, Iffland, 1993, Iffland et al., 1994). With prolonged alcoholization, methanol even rises beyond the maximum absorbed value (Figure 6, wine). The reason is that every human has endogenous methanol with levels of 0, 95 mg/l on an average as we found in than 508 sober subjects, independent of gender, age or body weight (Figure 4, Gilg, 1992, Haffner et al., 1996, 1997c, 1998). Thinking of the competitive inhibition by ethanol it was to be expected that not only absorbed, but also preexisting systemic, endogenous methanol will accumulate in the organism. It was clearly demonstrated that an ethanol load without any methanol or other possible methanol sources (like fruit) lead to a build-up and rise of endogenous methanol (Gilg et al., 1987b). According to experiments with isolated perfused rat liver and other investigations the origine of endogenous methanol seems to be based on biochemical metabolism (Gilg et al., 1987a), linked to a reduction of formaldehyde and the monocarbon resp. folate metabolism with S-adenosylmethionine / homocystein. A colonic bacterial activity cannot be ruled out, a dietary source seems to be occasional. Only gross amounts of fruits, fruit juice or pectines (with methylesters) may lead to elevated methanol levels (Gilg, 1989, Gilg, 1995, Lindinger et al., 1997), apart from inhalation or dermal resorption of methanol. As we found and proposed, the origine of endogenous methanol is much more supposed to be the intermediary metabolism than a dietary intake through food or an activity of intestinal flora. We found low over all contents in the stomach and slightly higher levels in lower intestines in autopsy cases (Gilg, 1992). In view of finding plant particles in the stool in the lower digestive tract, this is more the result of pectin break down than of bacterial fermentation. Methanol is not a direct product of fermentation, but derives from methylesters in pectin of fruits and plants. This explains high levels as seen in fruit brandy. Elevated methanol levels in blood may result after intake of fruit or fruit juice, but only if consumed in gross amounts. Normal consumption of fruits like two apples leads to minor methanol levels, only gross amounts like 10 bananas - which remind more on an animal than a human experiment - may result in relevant and quasi false positive levels. Pure vegetarians may reach 9 mg / l (but are not supposed to abuse alcohol).

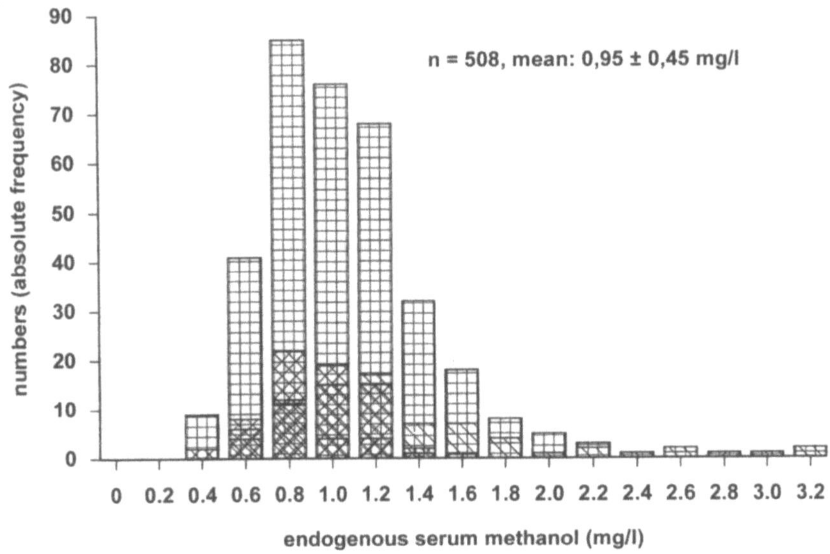

Figure 4 Endogenous serum methanol in 508 subjects (with no differencies in gender, healthy subjects, children, alcoholics and hepatopathies of different origine)

Figure 5 summarizes principles of the accumulation of merely endogenous methanol under ethanol in 50 subjects without recent alcohol consumption (Gilg, 1992, Gilg, 1995). The averaged build up of endogenous methanol is 0, 27 mg / l per hour. After consumption of red wine in a single experiment, this accumulation is effective and representative beyond the terminal state of methanol absorption. Based on calculations the rise of methanol seems to be limited by compensating physical elimination through sweat, urine, or breath, if levels reach a steady state with appr. 10 mg /l. Therefore even in chronic alcoholics with days of more or less persisting alcoholization resp. elevated methanol, methanol needs not to reach higher resp. toxic levels. The highest SMC we found and which is reported in literature was 180 mg/ l. Levels exceeding 50 mg/l are mostly combined with a recent or former consumption of fruit brandy.

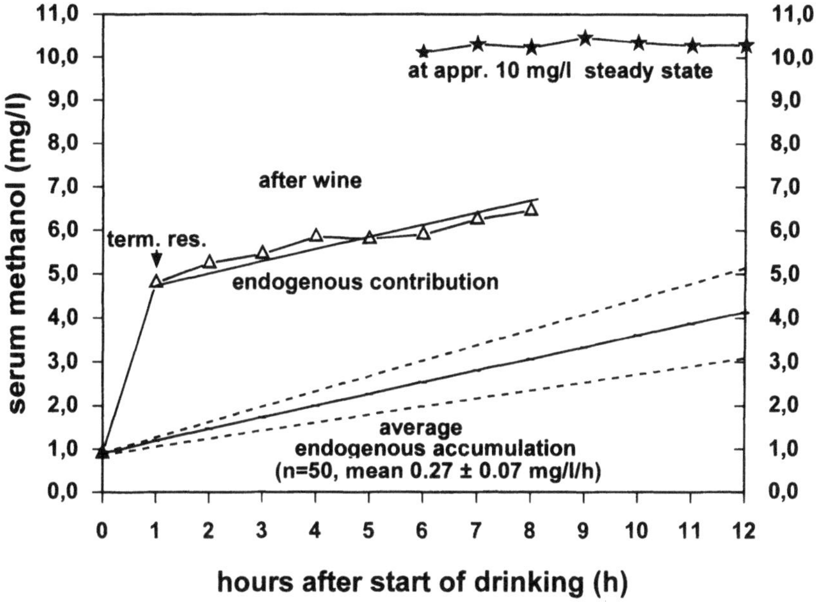

Figure 5 Accumulation of endogenous serum methanol under ethanol, compared to absorbed methanol of close to 5 mg/l after consumption of wine with subsequent accumulation of endogenous methanol. No further accumulation after appr. 10 mg/l serum methanol are reached.

This effect is also verifiable - by the way - if 4 - methylpyrazolone (4 - MP, now available as fomezipole) is taken, which is an effective ADH - blocker (alcohol dehydrogenase blocker). Figure 6 shows, that after bolus consumption of pure fruit brandy, quite high SMC may result, which persist as long as inhibiting ethanol levels are present. The same effect happens with 4 - MP, if taken initially in combination with fruit brandy or also if 4 – MP is taken at a blood alcohol of 0, 2 ‰. 4 - MP taken alone also leads to an endogenous build up of methanol. 4 - MP therefore can be used as an antidote in methanol intoxications. Furthermore possible effects of 4 - MP taken during withdrawal would be interesting, especially in view of effects of methanol on the metabolism of monocarbons, which is not investigated so far.

What are the practical consequences of elevated SMC? From a statistical view, we have a coincidence of elevated methanol and higher BAC in drunk drivers (Figure 4, other reports).

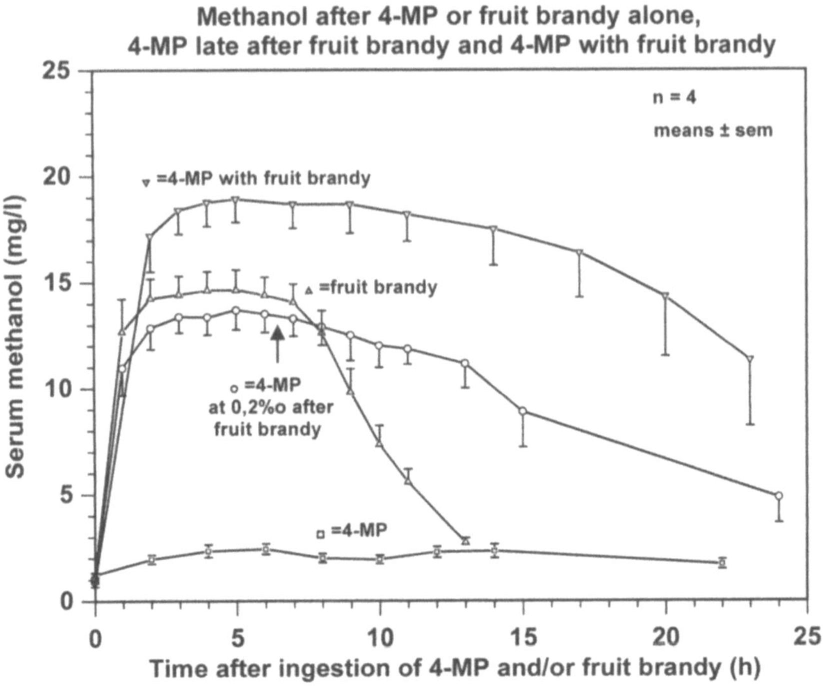

Figure 6 Methanol after consumption of fruit brandy alone, with 4-Methylpyrazol (4-MP) initially and during drinking. 4-MP also causes an accumulation of endogenous methanol.

By the way, this underlines, that we have more to deal with driving drinkers than with drunk drivers. The BAC of sentenced drunk drivers in Germany is 1, 6 to 1, 7 ‰ on an average since years. Generally it is widely accepted that serum methanol > 10 mg/l (or 8mg/l in blood) can only be achieved by prolonged periods of alcoholization resp. heavier drinking (Barz, 1993, Grüner and Bilzer, 1985, Iffland et al., 1984, 1989, Iffland and Staak, 1990, Iffland, 1993, Iffland et al., 1994).

The elimination of methanol is limited to BAC well below 0, 5 or even 0, 2 or 0 ‰, in alcoholics as well as in healthy and non abusing consumers. Concentration - time curves were taken from an alcoholic during withdrawal and clearly show this (Figure 8 and 9), supported by other reports (Bilzer et al., 1991, Haffner et al., 1993, 1997a,b, Jones and Sternebring, 1992). A unique report in the literature on an elimination of methanol in the presence of ethanol only in alcoholics is not convincing and questionable, also it is in contradiction to results of 5 other research groups (Musshoff et al, 1995).

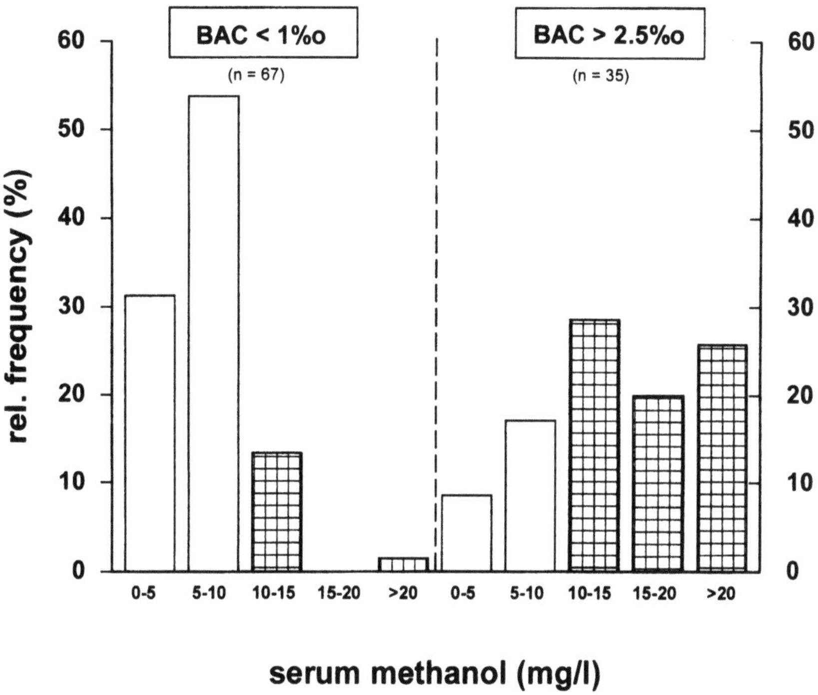

Figure 7 Relative frequency of serum methanol in drunken drivers with BAC < 1 ‰ and > 2.5 ‰

Figure 8 gives an additional overview on methanol characteristics in alcoholics during withdrawal with initial SMC lower than 50 mg/l (semilogarithmic), figure 9 presents the remaining three cases in this study with up to 140 mg/L (linear). Comparing linear and semilogarithmic elimination following the method of least square clearly shows an exponential elimination in all 13 cases following Michaelis - Menten kinetics. The mean half time is appr. 2, 4 hours (comparable to other consecutive studies, Haffner et al., 1993, 1997a,b). For rough estimations,

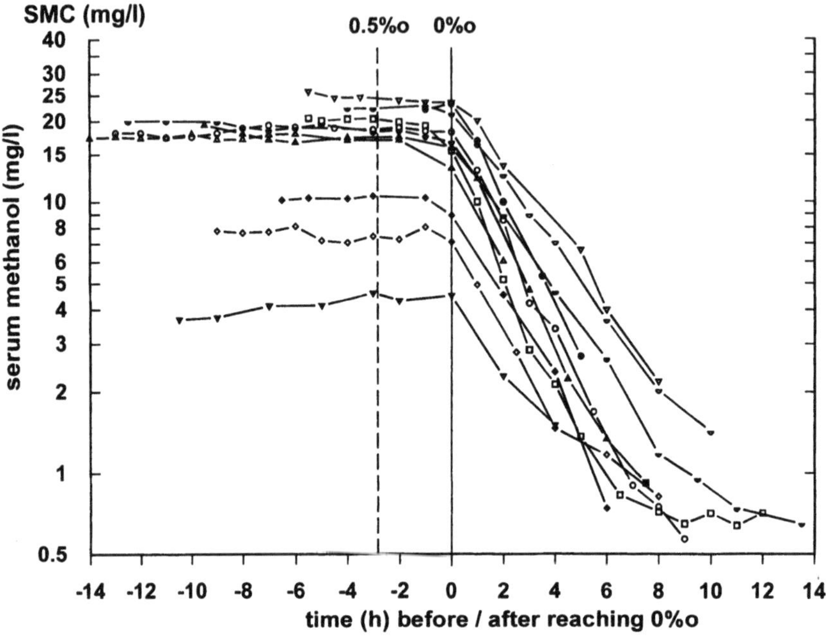

Figure 8 Serum methanol during withdrawal (semilogarithmic, initial values < 40 mg/l)

one could also apply a linear elimination with 4 mg /l per hour. This means, that it sometimes takes many hours to clear methanol even after terminal elimination of ethanol. Finding elevated SMC in absence of BAC can give valuable information not only on former and longer alcoholisation, but also allows to judge the risk of a - possibly fatal - withdrawal or epileptic fit, e.g. in autopsy or intensive care cases. Figure 10 shows details of one subject including acetone, with a coincidence of elevated acetone and severity of withdrawal symptoms resp. epileptic fit. Reasons and biochemical relations are unclear and should be evaluated in further studies. Also methanol may be related to withdrawal or hangover symptoms, as presented by Prof. Jones in this volume. It has to be clarified if this is based merely on the longer and heavier alcohol abuse or if it is a specific effect of methanol resp. formaldehyde. There are speculative reports on S-adenosylmethionine being involved in methanol metabolism as well as a hyperformaldehydism in schizophrenia (Andreoli and Maffei, 1975, Barker et al., 1980). Additional experiments are required to clarify, if formaldehyde, deriving from methanol in

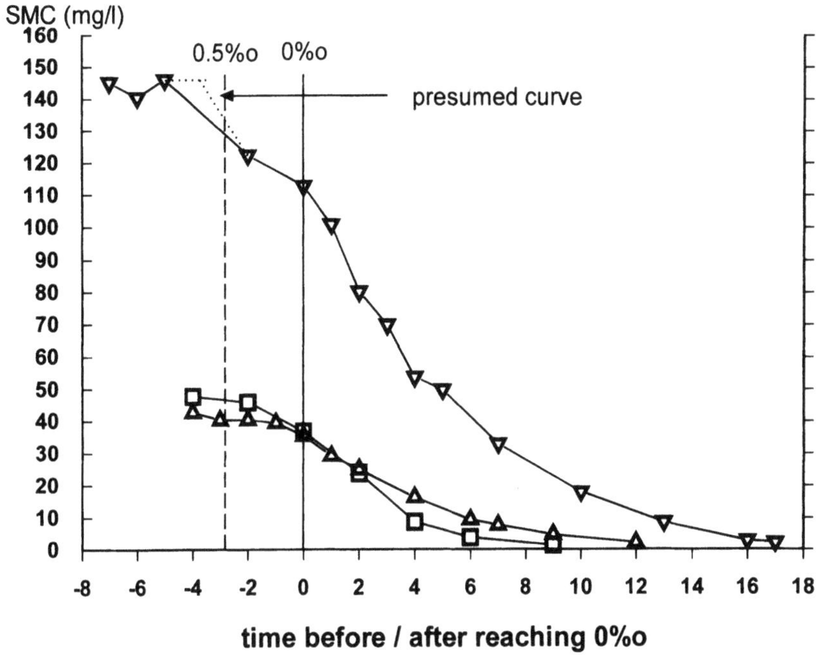

Figure 9 Serum methanol during withdrawal in 3 cases with initial levels > 40 mg/l. (numeric, the sampling interval of 3 hours may point at an elimination of methanol with ethanol > 0,5 ‰, which cannot be verified)

this phase, and a possible build up of tetrahydroisoquinolines (TIQ) are relevant. Also the influence of methanol on the C1 - metabolism may be relevant (e.g. there is a linkage to homocystein as a risk factor for atherosclerosis, to DNA changes and a higher risk for cancer in alcoholics or folate deficiencies, Wu et al., 1975), especially in view of the development and course of alcohol dependence or subsequent illnesses resp. organ disturbances.

Acetone shows an interesting curve in figure 10 as well as in other subjects of the study, especially in view of an epileptic fit happening after the elevation and during the descending part. Acetone exceeding 7 mg /l is mainly the result of disturbed ketone metabolism, as through starvation, hypothermia or diabetic or alcoholic ketosis and can give valuable diagnostic information, e.g. in autopsy cases in view of alcoholic ketoacidosis (Fulop et al., 1986). If the effect in the example is specific to withdrawal or a reduction of carbohydrate intake or indicating the degree and severity of withdrawal symptoms is still not clear. Elevated acetone levels may also derive from starvation, freezing and diabetic ketosis.

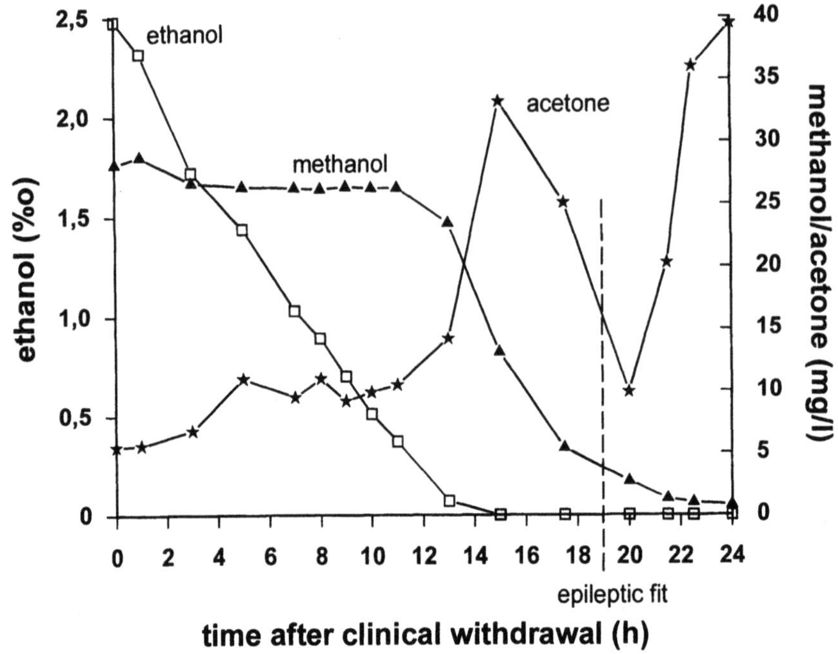

Figure 10 Ethanol, methanol and acetone during withdrawal

Additionally, isopropanol levels exceeding 2 mg/l or summarized values of isopropanol + acetone of more than 9 mg/L are regarded as similar markers (Davis et al., 1984, Gilg, 1992, 1995, Iffland and Staak, 1990, Inoue, 1984). Isopropanol is not a constituent of alcoholic beverages, but derives from acetone during ethanol metabolism, which leads to an elevated redox potential resp. NADH (reduction of acetone to isopropanol by ADH and NADH) and a shift from acetone to isopropanol. During withdrawal and without ethanol, isopropanol is oxidized to acetone and not detectable any more. Elevated levels of acetone and isopropanol indicate recent alcohol abuse, possibly combined with reduced nourishment.

Finally figure 11 shows basic parameters of methanol and figure 12 gives an overview on time characteristics of classical and newer markers of alcohol abuse (overviews on markers in: Bendtsen et al., 1998, Gilg et al., 1995, Gilg, 1999, Pullarkat and Simhachalam, 1985, Stamm et al., 1993, Thomas, 1998). They represent various biochemical reactions on alcohol abuse, mainly based on enzymatic inhibition and side effects and usually show no (quantitative) correlations. An evaluation of alcohol markers to this respect may be helpful to identify different drinking habits (unless non responders have to be considered).

BASICS FOR EVALUATIONS AND CALCULATIONS WITH METHANOL

Mean endogenous serum methanol:	app.1 ± 0,5mg/l
Widmark value for expected serum levels:	r = 0,6
Endogenous cumulation under ethanol (>0,5‰):	app. 0,3 ± 0,1mg/l
Steady-state methanol under ethanol (>0,5‰):	app. 8-10mg/l
Lack of relevant systemic methanol elimination in healthy subjects and alcoholics	BAC >0,5‰
methanol elimination with ethanol lower 0,5 - 0‰ mean half time	2,4 ± 0,5 Stunden

Figure 11 Basic parameters for evaluation and calculations of methanol

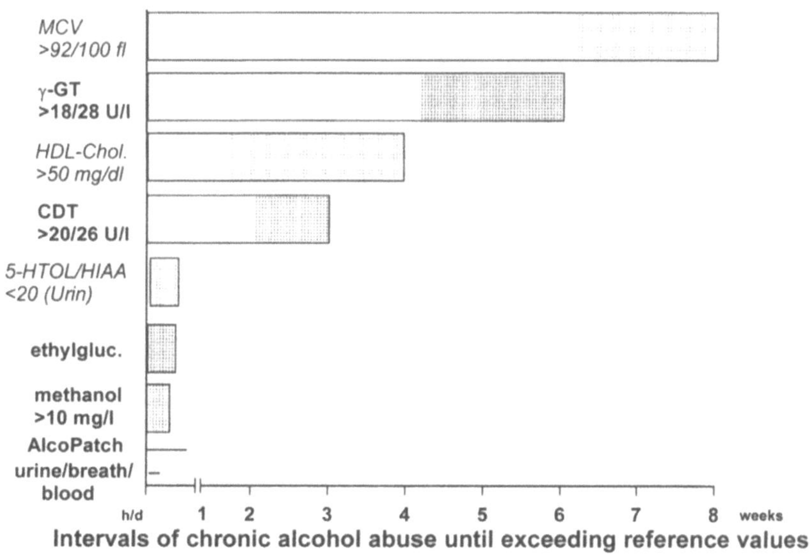

Figure 12 Comparison of different markers for alcohol abuse in view of time intervals until reacting resp. exceeding reference values

References

Andreoli VM., Maffei F., Letter: Blood-levels of S-adenosylmethionine in schizophrenia, Lancet 79, 922 (1975).

Barker SA., Carl GF., Monti JA., Hyperformaldehydism: A unifying hypothesis for the major biochemical theories of schizophrenia, Med Hypotheses 6, 671-686 (1980).

Barz J., Zum Nachweis des chronischen Alkoholmißbrauchs bei alkoholisierten Verkehrsteilnehmern (Review), Zbl Rechtsmed 39, 623-628 (1993).

Bendtsen P., Jones AW., Helander A., Urinary excretion of methanol and 5-hydroxytryptophol as biochemical markers of recent drinking in the hangover state, Alcohol Alcohol 33, 431-439 (1998).

Bilzer N., Schmutte P., Jehs M., Penners BM., Kinetik aliphatischer Alkohole (Methanol, Propanol-1 und Isobutanol) bei Anwesenheit von Äthanol im menschlichen Körper, Blutalkohol 27, 385-409 (1990).

Bilzer N., Penners BM., Conrad A., Methanolkinetic in alcoholics, Blutalkohol 28, 377-392 (1991).

Bonte W., Hey F., Zur Frage der Lagerungsveränderungen von Begleitstoffbefunden in Blut- und Urinproben Blutalkohol 20, 109-122 (1983).

Bonte W., Begleitstoffe alkoholischer Getränke, Schmidt-Römhild Verlag, (1987).

Bonte W., Sprung R., Lesch OM., Neue biochemische Überlegungen zur Suchtentwicklung, Wien Z Suchtforsch 11, 15-18 (1988).

Bonte W., Barz J., Lesch OM., Formaldehyde and its possible role in chronic alcoholism, Alc Drugs Traffic Safety, Heft 3, 3298 (1991).

Collins MA., Methanol as a marker of alcohol abuse (letter), Alcohol Clin Exp Res 14, 633 (1990).

Davis PL., Dal LA., Cortivo D., Maturo J., Endogenous Isopropanol: Forensic and Biochemical implications, J Anal Toxicol 8, 209-212 (1984).

DiPadova C., Alderman J., Lieber CS., Improved methods for the measurement of acetaldehyde, concentrations in plasma and red blood cells, Alcohol Clin Exp Res 10, 86 (1986).

Eriksson CJ., Problems and pitfalls in acetaldehyde determinations, Alcohol Clin Exp Res 4, 22 (1980).

Eriksson CJ., Human blood acetaldehyde concentration during ethanol oxidation (Update 1982), Pharmacol Bioch Beh 18/S 1, 141-150 (1983).

Fischer G., Kampmann H., Verteilung exogenen Acetaldehyds im menschlichen Blut und deren, Beeinflußung durch Disulfiram, Blutalkohol 19, 447-458 (1982).

Fulop M., Ben-Ezra J., Bock J., Alcoholic ketosis, Alcohol Clin Exp Res 10, 610-615 (1986).

Gilg T., Nachweis von Begleitstoffen in alkoholischen Getränken, in Blut und Körperflüssigkeiten und deren Bedeutung, Med Welt 37, 246-248 (1986).

Gilg T., v.Meyer L., Liebhardt E., Schwabe U., Scholz R., Methanolbildung in der perfundierten Rattenleber beim Fremdstoffabbau unter Äthanolbelastung Blutalkohol 24, 316-320 (1987).

Gilg T., v. Meyer L., Liebhardt L., Zur Bildung und Akkumulation von endogenem Methanol unter Äthanolbelastung Blutalkohol 24, 321-332 (1987).

Gilg T., Soyka M., v. Meyer L., Ora I., Methanol und Iso-Propanol als biochemische Alkoholismusmarker, Psychiatrische und forensische Aspekte, Nervenheilkunde 8, 105-113 (1989).

Gilg T., Methanol: Stoffwechsel bei kurzzeitiger und chronischer Alkoholaufnahme und Stellenwert als biochemischer Alkoholismusmarker, Habilitationsschrift LMU-München, (1992).

Gilg T., Alkohol (Ethanol): Pharmakologie, BAK-Berechnung und forensische Begutachtung. In: Soyka M: Die Alkoholkrankheit-Diagnose und Therapie, Chapman and Hall, London- Glasgow-Weinheim, 18-104 (1995).

Gilg T., Deinl I., Grundner H., Soyka M., Stellenwert von Begleitstoffanalytik (Methanol, Isopropanol) und CD-Transferrin (CDT) in der Alkoholismusdiagnostik, In: Biologische Alkoholismusmarker (Hrsg.: M. Soyka), Chapman & Hall, Weinheim, London, Glasgow, S 45 – 92 (1995).

Gilg, T., Forensische Aspekte von Alkohol und Alkoholismus, In: Alkohol und Alkoholfolgekrankheiten, Hrsg. M. Singer, S. Teyssen, Kapitel 39, S 527 – 551 (1999), Springer-Verlag, Berlin-Heidelberg-New York.

Greenberg LA., The appearance of some congeners and their metabolites in blood, Quart J Stud Alcohol/S 5, 20-25 (1970).

Grüner O, Bilzer N., Blut-Methanol-Konzentrationen nach Genuß von Wodka, Blutalkohol 19, 459-464 (1982).

Grüner O., Bilzer N., Zur Teilnahme chronischer Alkoholiker am Straßenverkehr, Blutalkohol 22, 209-223 (1985).

Grüner O., Bilzer N., Liebmann J., Methanolbildung bei Pektingaben, Unfall- und Sicherheitsforschung im Straßenverkehr 89, 20-21, (1993).

Haffner HT., Batra A., Wehner HD., Besserer K., Mann K., Methanol levels and methanol elimination in alcoholics, Blutalkohol 30, 52-61 (1993).

Haffner HT., Graw M., Besserer K., Blickle U., Henssge C., Endogenous methanol: variability in concentration and rate of production. Evidence of a deep compartment?, Forensic Sci Int 79, 145-154 (1996).

Haffner HT., Besserer K., Graw M., Voges S., Methanol elimination in non-alcoholics: inter- and intraindividual variation, Forensic Sci Int 86, 69-76 (1997).

Haffner HT., Banger M., Graw M., Besserer K., Brink T., The kinetics of methanol elimination in alcoholics and the influence of ethanol, Forensic Sci Int 89, 129-136 (1997).

Haffner HT., Banger M., Graw M., Besserer K., Endogenous methanol production and methanol excretion in alcoholics, Blutalkohol 34, 270-275 (1997).

Haffner HT., Graw M., Besserer K., Stränger J., Curvilinear increase in methanol concentration after inhibition of oxidation by ethanol: significance for the investigation of endogenous methanol concentration and formation, Int J Legal Med 111, 27-31 (1998).

Hillman RS., Steinberg SE, The effects of alcohol on folate metabolism, Ann Rev Med 33, 345-354 (1982).

Iffland R., Kaschade W., Heesen D., Mehne P., Untersuchungen zur Bewertung hoher Methanolspiegel bei Begleitalkohol-Analysen, Beitr Ger Med 42, 231-236 (1984).

Iffland R., Balling P., Oehmichen M., Lieder F., Norpoth Th., Methanol, Isopropanol, n-Propanol - endogene Bildung unter Äthanoleinfluß?, Blutalkohol 26, 87-97 (1989).

Iffland R., Staak M., Methanol und Isopropanol als Alkoholismusmarker, Beitr Ger Med 48, 173-177 (1990).

Iffland R., CDT, GGT und Methanol als Alkoholismusindikatoren in Blutproben alkoholauffälliger Kraftfahrer, Fortschr Diagnost 4, Praxisreport 5, 17-22 (1993).

Iffland R., Balling P., Börsch G. et al., Zur Wertung erhöhter Spiegel von GGT, CDT, Methanol, Aceton und Isopropanol im Blut alkoholauffälliger Kraftfahrer , Alkoholismusindikatoren anstelle medizinisch-psychologischer Untersuchungen?, Blutalkohol 31/5, 287-314 (1994).

Inoue K., Fukunaga M., Kiriyama T., Komura S., Accumulation of acetaldehydes in alcohol-sensitive Japanese, Reaction to ethanol and acetaldehyde oxidizing capacity, Alcohol Clin Exp Res 8, 319-323 (1984).

Jones AW., Abnormally high concentrations of methanol in breath, A useful biochemical marker of recent heavy drinking, Clin Chem 32, 1241-1242 (1986).

Jones AW., Skagerberg S., Löwinger H., Occurence of methanol in blood and breath after administration of ethanol, Alcoholic beverage congener or raised concentration of an endogenous metabolite?, Proc Intern Workshop on Congeners of Alc Bev (Düsseldorf), 1987, 173-182 (1987).

Jones AW., Elimination half life of methanol during hangover, Pharmacol Toxicol 60, 217-220 (1987).

Jones AW., Löwinger H., Relationship between the concentration of ethanol and methanol in blood samples from swedish drinking drivers, For Sci Int 37, 277-285 (1988).

Jones AW., Skaggerberg S., Yonekura A., Sato A., Metabolic interaction between methanol and exogenous ethanol studied in human volunteers by analysis of breath, Pharmacol Toxicol 65, 48-53 (1989).

Jones AW., Sternebring B., Kinetics of ethanol and methanol in alcoholics during detoxification, Alcohol Alcoholism 27/6, 641-647 (1992).

Jones AW., Helander A., Changes in the concentrations of ethanol, methanol and metabolites of serotonin in two successive urinary voids from drinking drivers, Forensic Sci Int 93, 127-134 (1998).

Korri UA., Nuutinen H., Salaspuro M., Increased blood acetate: A new laboratory marker of alcoholism and heavy drinking, Alcohol Clin Exp Res 9, 468-471 (1985).

Lands WEM., Acetate metabolism: New mysteries from old data, Alcohol Clin Exp Res 15, 393-394 (1991).

Lindinger W., Taucher J., Jordan A., Hansel A., Vogel W., Endogenous production of methanol after the consumption of fruit, Alcoholism Clin Exp Res 21, 939-943 (1997).

Machata G., Prokop L. Über Begleitsubstanzen alkoholischer Getränke im Blut, Blutalkohol 8, 349-353 (1971).

Magrinat G., Ethanol and methanol metabolites in alcohol withdrawal, Nature 244, 234-235 (1973).

Majchrowicz E., Mendelson JH., Blood concentrations of acetaldehyde and ethanol in chronic alcoholics, Science 168, 1100-1102 (1970).
Majchrowicz E., Sutherland VC., Detection and identification of methanol in urine of drinking alcoholics, Pharmacologist 13, 219 (1971).
Majchrowicz E., Mendelson JH., Blood methanol concentrations during experimentally induced ethanol intoxication in alcoholics, J Pharmacol Exp Therap 179, 293-300 (1971).
Majchrowicz E., Steinglass P., Blood methanol, blood ethanol and alcohol withdrawal syndrome in humans, Fed Proc 32, 728 (1973).
Majchrowicz E. Metabolic correlates of ethanol, acetaldehyde, acetate and methanol in humans and animals, Adv Exp Med Biol 56, 111-140 (1975).
Meyer HJ., Gilg T.., v. Meyer L., Methanol in Blutproben nach Lagerung und bakterieller Beimpfung, Zbl Rechtsmed 42/6, 443 (1994).
Musshoff F., Daldrup T., Bonte W., Leitner A., Nimmerrichter A., Walter H., Lesch OM., Ethanolunabhängige Methanolelimination bei chronischen Alkoholikern, Blutalkohol 32, 317-336 (1995).
Nykänen L., Suomalainen H., Aroma of beer, wine and distilled alcoholic beverages, D. Reidel Publishing Company, 20-22 (1983).
Nykänen L., Suomalainen H., Occurence of methyl alcohols, Handbuch der Aromaforschung, Akademie Verlag, Berlin, (1983).
Peschel O., Bauer MF., Gilg T., v.Meyer L., Veränderung von Begleitstoffanalysen durch percutane Resorption, propanolhaltiger Antiseptika, Blutalkohol 29, 172-184 (1992).
Pieper WA., Skeen MJ., Changes in blood methanol concentrations in chimpanzees during periods of chronic ethanol ingestion, Biochem Pharmacol 22, 163-173 (1973).
Pullarkat RK., Simhachalam R., Elevated urinary dolichol levels in chronic alcoholics, Alcohol Clin Exp Res 9, 28 (1985).
Rietbrock N., Kinetik und Wege des Methanolumsatzes, Arch Pharmakol Exp Path 263, 88-105 (1969).
Roe O., Species differences in methanol poisoning, CRC Crit Rev Toxicol 10, 275-290 (1982).
Roine RP., Eriksson CJP., Ylikahri R. et al, Methanol as a Marker of Alcohol Abuse, Alcohol Clin Exp Res 13, 172-175 (1989).
Sprung R., Bonte W., Lesch OM., Methanol, Ein bisher verkannter Bestandteil aller alkoholischen Getränke, Eine neue biochemische Annäherung an das Problem des chronischen Alkoholismus, Wien Klin Wochenschr 100, 282-288 (1988).
Sprung R., Bonte W., Die Bedeutung der sogenannten Begleitstoffe für Suchtentwicklung und Spätschäden des chronischen Alkoholismus, Wien Z Suchtforsch 11, 19-24 (1988).
Stamm D., Hansert E., Feuerlein W., Excessive consumption of alcohol in men as a biological influence factor in clinical laboratory investigations, J. Clin Chem Clin Biochem 22, 65-77 (1984), Acta Neurol Scand 88/4, 279-283 (1993).
Stöhlmacher P., Zur Bildung sogenannter Begleitstoffe (Propanole, Butanole u.a.) aus Ethanol durch Mikroorganismen, Blutalkohol 33, 113-141 (1996).
Tsokos M., Grüner O., Bilzer N., Penners BM., Methanol kinetics under treatment with the H2-antagonist ranitidine, Blutalkohol 33, 267-280 (1996).
Thomas L. (Hrsg), Labor und Diagnose, Die medizinische Verlagsgruppe, Marburg (1998).
Wargotz ES., Werner M., Asymptomatic blood methanol in emergency room patients, Am J. Clin Pathol 87, 773-775 (1987).
Wu A., Chanarin I., Slavin G., Levi AJ., Folate deficiency in the alcoholic-its relationship to clinical and haematological abnormalities, liver disease and folate stores, Br J. Haematol 29, 469-478 (1975).

5-HTOL is a sensitive marker of recent alcohol consumption

Stefan Borg
Olof Beck*

Stefan Borg
Karolinska Institute
Dept of Clinical Neurosciences
Beroendecentrum Nord
Box 125 60
102 29 Stockholm
Sweden

Dept of Clinical Pharmacology*
Karolinska Hospital
Stockholm
Sweden

Phone: +46-8-672 1451
FAX: +46-8-672 1904
Email: stefan.borg@cspo.sll.se

Biochemical background

Increased 5-hydroxytryptophol (5-HTOL) – a natural constituent of human urine - can be used as a marker of recent alcohol consumption. It is formed in the body as a metabolite of serotonin (5-hydroxytryptamine, or 5-HT) and is excreted in urine after conjugation with glucuronic acid (Bosin, 1978). The catabolic pathway of serotonin consists of oxidative deamination to 5-hydroxyindole-3-acetaldehyde (5-HIAL) by the enzyme monoamine oxidase (EC1.4.3.4). 5-HIAL is then either oxidazed by aldehyde dehydrogenase (EC 1.2.1.3) to form 5-hydroxyindole-3-acetic acid (5-HIAA) or reduced by alcohol dehydrogenase (EC 1.1.1.1) or aldehyde reductase (EC 1.1.1.2) to form 5-HTOL, see figure 1.

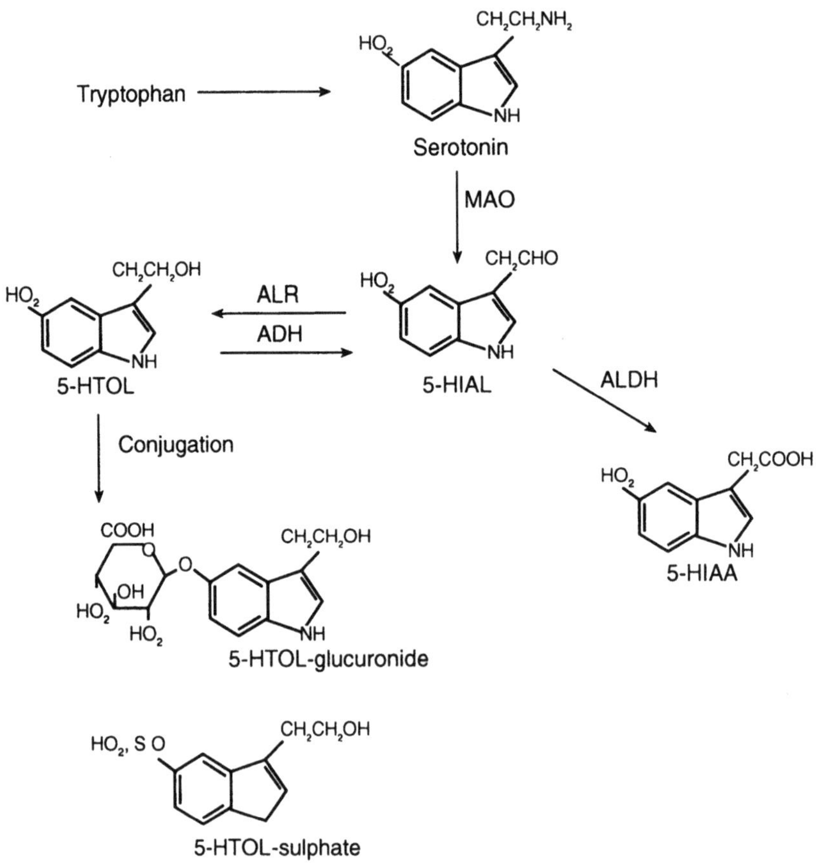

Figure 1 Serotonin metabolism. Serotonin is formed in two steps from the essential amino acid tryptophan. The first catabolic step of serotonin is oxidation by monoamine oxidase (MAO) to 5-hydroxyindoleacetaldehyde (5-HIAL). This intermediate aldehyde is either oxidized by aldehyde dehydrogenase (ALDH) to 5-hydroxyindoleacetic acid (5-HIAA), or reduced by alcohol

dehydrogenase (ADH) or aldehyde reductase (ARL) to 5-hydroxytryptophol (5-HTOL). The urinary excretion of 5-HTOL is facilitated by formation of glucuronide and sulphate conjugate.

Normally, 5-HIAA is by far the most abundant end product of 5-HT metabolism, >95 % (Beck et.al., 1984). However, the catabolism is altered shortly after alcohol intake, resulting in decreased formation of 5-HIAA and a concomitant dose-dependent increase in 5-HTOL. 5-HTOL may constitute as much as 50 % of total serotonin metabolism. This effect is suggested to be the result of either competitive inhibition of aldehyde dehydrogenase by the ethanol-derived acetaldehyde or the increased ratio between NADH and NAD+, both of which favour reduction of 5-HIAL to 5-HTOL (Walsh, 1973).

The shift toward the reductive pathway is observable in the urine several hours after the ethanol has disappeared from the body, see figure 2 (Beck et al., 1984) Based on these findings, increased urinary excretion of 5-HTOL has been proposed as a promising diagnostic marker of recent alcohol consumption in the treatment of alcohol dependence.

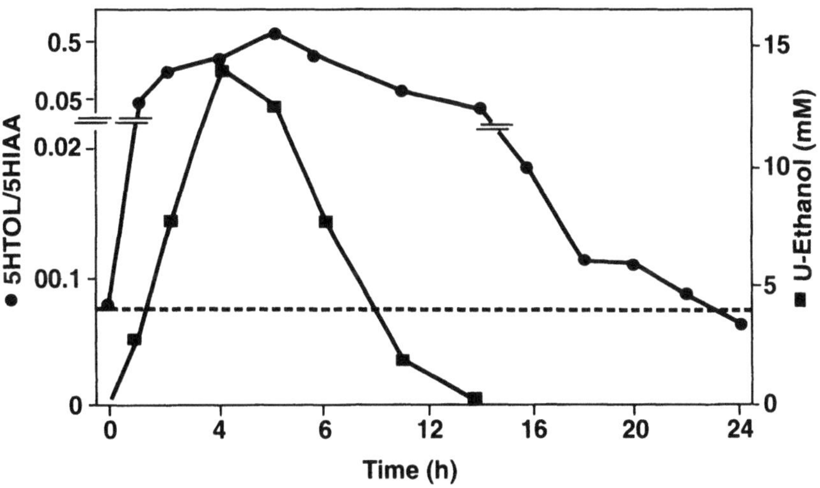

Figure 2 Urinary 5-HTOL / 5-HIAA ratio after acute ethanol intake (0,8g/kg) in healthy volunteers. The increase in 5-HTOL / 5-HIAA is present longer than ethanol is detected.

Analytical methods

Urinary 5-HTOL (free + conjugated form) has been determined by a sensitive and specific gas chromatographic-mass spectrometric (GC-MS) method. (Beck et al., 1980) One important improvement that has been made is the use of bacterial β-glucuronidase for the hydrolysis of conjugated 5-HTOL. With the new enzyme, the hydrolysis is performed in 1 hour as opposed to 16 with the previously used enzyme from Helix pomatia (sulfatase type H-1). However, mass spectrometric methods are not optimal when large numbers of samples are to be analyzed in clinical routine. Therefore, a simple and reproducible high-performance liquid chromatography (HPLC) method for the determination of elevated urinary levels of 5-HTOL has been developed. (Helander et al., 1991) This method is probably more suitable for use in clinical laboratory screening. In brief, a 20-μL sample was hydrolyzed for 1 h at 37°C using β-glucuronidase. A centrifuged aliquot was then diluted with ice-cold deionized water and injected directly into an isocratically eluted Nucleosil C18 reversed-phase column.

Alternatively, 5-HTOL was isolated by one-step sample cleanup procedure on a small Sephadex G10 column prior to HPLC analysis. After the sample cleanup, no major interfering peaks were observed in the chromatograms. Presence of 5-HTOL was determined by electrochemical detection (+ 0.60 V vs Ag/AgCl reference). A good correlation (r2 = 0.97) was obtained between the HPLC method and the GC-MS method when analyses were performed on urine samples containing 200 - 2500 pmol/mL of 5-HTOL. The intraassay coefficients of variation with a 5-HTOL standard containing 1000 pmol/mL and a urine sample containing 1800 pmol/mL were 1.4 and 1.7 %, respectively (n = 6). In urine (as a conjugate), 5-HTOL was stable for at least 12 months when stored at –20 or -80°C.

Clinical characteristics

Since the 5-HTOL excretion does not return to normal until several hours after the blood and urinary ethanol levels have reached zero (Beck et al., 1982), an increased urinary level of 5-HTOL can be used as a sensitive biochemical marker to indicate recent alcohol consumption (Voltaire et al 1992).

For routine clinical use, urinary 5-HTOL is preferably expressed relative to 5-HIAA instead of creatinine, since ingestion of foods rich in 5-HT (e.g., bananas, pineapple, kiwi, tomatoes, and walnuts) could otherwise yield false-positive results. (Helander et al., 1992, Helander et al., 1994) This also contributes to increased sensitivity of the marker, since 5-HTOL increases at the expense of 5-HIAA during ethanol metabolism.

The limit to discriminate between normal and elevated levels of the 5-HTOL/5-HIAA ratio was originally set at 20 pmol/nmol (Voltaire et al., 1992). At this limit, the probability of having a positive outcome in the test during abstinence from alcohol was calculated to be less than 0.001. (Voltaire et al., 1992) In a group of four volunteers drinking over 200 g of ethanol a week, more than 50 % of the urine samples collected during a 3-months period were greater than 0.02 in the 5-HTOL/5-HIAA assay.

In a more careful study of a larger number of abstinent subjects of both Caucasian and Oriental origin, a lower cut-off limit of 15 pmol/nmol could be introduced (Helander et al., 1994). The within-day and day-to-day stability during periods of abstinence has been found to be very high (Voltaire et al., 1992). Both 5-HTOL and 5-HIAA are relatively stable in urine samples upon handling and storage (Helander et al., 1991, Helander et al., 1992).

Since urinary 5-HTOL does not return to baseline level until several hours after ethanol is no longer detectable, the sensitivity of 5-HTOL to detect recent alcohol consumption is superior to measurement of ethanol in clinical settings. In an experiment where healthy subjects drank moderate amounts of alcohol (3 - 98 g/day, mean 25 g), 52 out of 77 drinking occasions were detected in the next by an elevated 5-HTOL level, but only 5 by presence of ethanol. The results for one subject are shown in figure 3.

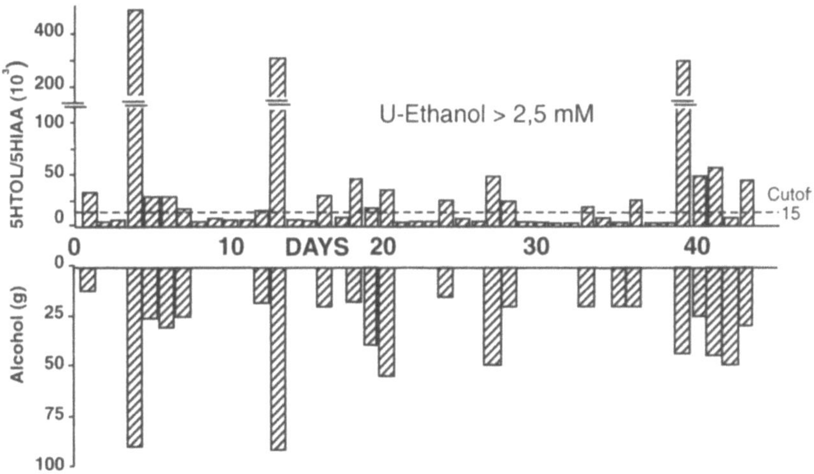

Figure 3 Record of ethanol intake and 5-HTOL / 5HIAA values in morning urine during one month in a non-alcoholic subject.

Genetic variation in ADH and ALDH did not influence the 5-HTOL/5-HIAA baseline level (Helander et al., 1994), despite the well-known modulatory effects on the degradation of ethanol. Hitherto, the only known factor other than alcohol consumption that may lead to an elevated (i.e. false-positive) 5-HTOL/5-HIAA ratio is treatment with drugs inhibiting the enzyme ALDH (disulfiram and cyanamide) (Beck et al., 1995). However, the response to ALDH inhibitors was less pronounced than the effect seen after ethanol intake. In fact, in some subjects, no effect at all on the 5-HTOL/5-HIAA ratio could be observed. The effect of disulfiram was more long-lasting than that of cyanamide.

The fact that intake of Disulfiram gave stable and small increase in 5-HTOL levels of urine can be used as an indication of an effective enzyme inhibition and thus a marker that the treatment is effective, either concerning dose range or compliance (Beck et al., 1995).

Furthermore, alcohol intake during Disulfiram treatment will give rise to even higher levels of 5-HTOL thus improving the possibilities to detect alcohol intake. (Beck et al 1995, Helander et al., 1998).

More than 20 patients have been followed during treatment with this marker. Examples from two patients are shown in figure 4. In the first patient (Figure 4 A), one occasion with an abnormal 5-HTOL to 5-HIAA ratio was detected, and the consumption of alcohol was verified clinically. In this patient, the stability of the 5-HTOL to 5-HIAA ratio during periods of abstinence from alcohol is apparent. In the other example (Figure 4 B), the patient had relapsed into regular alcohol consumption, which was revealed by elevated 5-HTOL to 5-HIAA ratios.

5-HTOL in urine is not formed after death. This fact has been used to differentiate between alcohol formed before and after death in forensic practise (Helander et al. 1992).

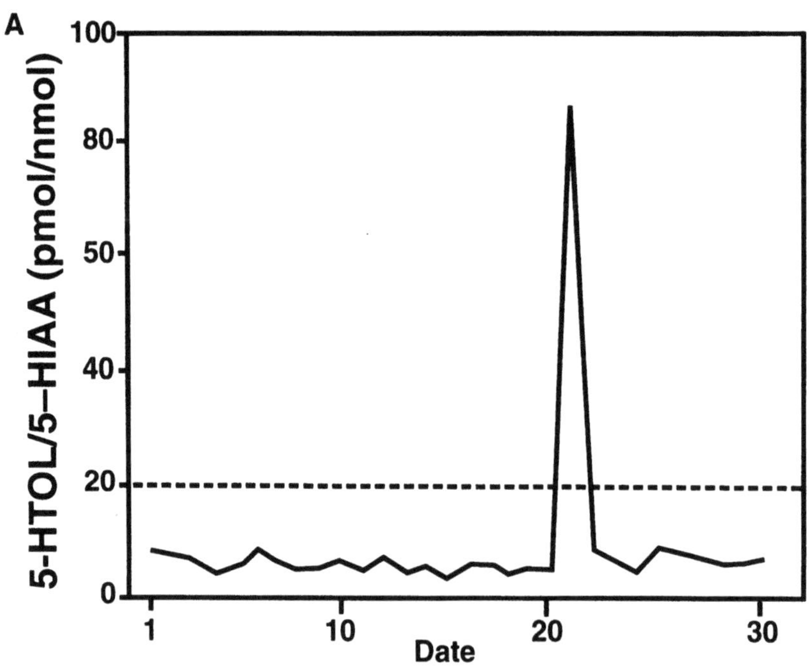

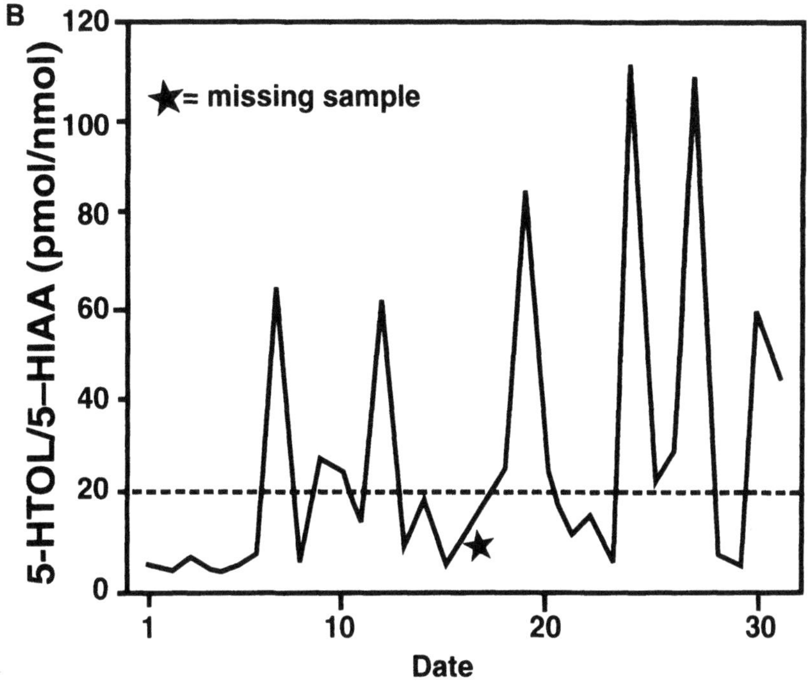

Figure 4 (A + B) The molar ratio of 5-HTOL to 5-HIAA x 1000 in urine from two alcoholic patients during treatment period of 1 mo.

Different markers are often compared concerning sensitivity and specificity. In a comparative study supported by ISBRA and WHO preliminary data confirmed the high specificity and sensitivity in comparison to other markers (Helander et al., 1997), despite the fact 5-HTOL should be seen as a marker of alcohol intake and not abuse or dependence.

It can even be used to detect relapse and lapses in alcohol dependent patients groups (Voltaire et al., 1992). As single lapses can be detected it is possible for the treatment staff to intervene before the simple lapse has developed to relapse and heavy alcohol consumption. By introducing 5-HTOL in relapse prevention improvement of treatment results could be expected.

Conclusions

5-HTOL has been shown to be a sensitive and specific marker of recent alcohol intake. Today methods based on GCMS and HPLC has been developed. By using the ratio of 5-HTOL/5-HIAA the problems with urine dilution and changes in overall serotonin metabolism can be managed and stable levels of HTOL determined in sample of urine. Single intakes of alcohol down to amounts as low as 20 - 25 g can be detected the day after.

The main area for use are

- detection of single lapses and relapses during treatment
- differential diagnosis in clinical praxis, e.g. trauma and emergency units
- control for compliance of Disulfiram treatment
- differentiating between alcohol intake before and after death in forensic practise
- control of single doses of alcohol intake in for instance work place and security programs

References

Beck O., Borg S., Eriksson L. and Lundman A.; 5-hydroxytryptophol in the cerebrospinal fluid and urine of alcoholics and healthy subjects. Naunyn-Schmiedebergs Arch Pharmacol, 321:293-297, 1982

Beck O., Borg S., Holmstedt B. and Stibler H.; Levels of 5-hydroxytryptophol in cerebrospinal fluid from alcoholics determined by gas chromatography-mass spectrometry. Biochemical Pharmacology, vol 29:693-696, 1980

Beck O., Borg S., Jonsson G., Lundman A. and Valverius P.; Measurement of 5-hydroxytryptophol and 5-hydroxyindoleacetic acid in human and rat brain and plasma. J Neuroal Transm, 59:57-67, 1984

Beck O., Helander A., Carlsson S.and Borg S.; Changes in serotonin metabolism during treatment with the aldehyde dehydrogenase inhibitors disulfiram and cyanamide. Pharmacology & Toxiclogy, 77:323-326, 1995

Bosin T. R.; Serotonin metabolism, Serotonin in Health and Disease, vol 1, W B Essman, ed. (Spectrum, New York), 181-300, 1978.

Helander A. and Tabakoff B.; WHO/ISBRA, Study Centres; Biochemical markers of alcohol use and abuse: Experiences from the pilot study of the WHO/ISBRA collaborative project on state and trait markers of alcohol. Alcohol Alcohol, 32:133-144, 1997.

Helander A., Beck O. and Borg S.; Determination of urinary 5-hydroxytryptophol by high-performance liquid chromatography with electrochemical detection. J Chromat, 579:340-345, 1992

Helander A., Beck O. and Jones W.; Urinary 5-HTOL/5-HIAA as biomedical marker of postmortem ethanol synthesis. Lancet 340:1159, 1992

Helander A., Beck O., Wennberg M., Wikström T. and Jacobsson G.; Determination of urinary 5-hydroxyindole-3-acetic acid by high-performance liquid chromatography with electrochemical detection and direct sample injection. Anal Biochem, 196:170-173, 1991.

Helander A., von Wachemfeldt J., Hiltunen A., Beck O., Liljeberg P. and Borg S.; Comparison of urinary 5-hydroxytryptophol, breath ethanol, and self-report for detection of recent alcohol use during outpatient treatment: A study on methadone patients. Drug and Alcohol Dependence, 56:33-38, 1999

Helander A., Walzer C., Beck O., Balant L., Borg S. and Wartburg J. P.; Influence of genetic variation in alcohol and aldehyde dehydrogenase on serotonin metabolism. Life Sci, 55:359-366, 1994.

Helander A., Wikström T., Löwenmo C., Jacobsson G. and Beck O.; Urinary excretion of 5-hydroxyindole-3-acetic acid and 5-hydroxytryptophol after oral loading with serotonin. Life Sci, 50:1207-1213, 1992

Helander A.; Monitoring relapse drinking during disulfiram therapy by assay of urinary 5-hydroxytryptophol. Alcohol Clin Exp Res, 22:111-114, 1998

Voltaire A. Carlsson S., Hiltunen A. J., Beck O., Stibler H. and Borg S.; Detection of relapses in alcohol-dependent patients: Comparison of carbohydrate deficient transferrin in serum, 5-hydroxytryptophol in urine and self-reports. Alcohol Clin Exp Res, 17:703-708, 1993.

Voltaire A., Beck O. and Borg S.; Urinary 5-hydroxytryptophol : A possible marker of recent alcohol consumption. Alcohol Clin Exp Res, 16:281-285, 1992

Walsh M. J.; Role of acetaldehyde in the interactions of ethanol with neuroamines. Adv Mental Sci, 3:233-266, 1973

The direct ethanol metabolite ethyl glucuronide: A specific marker of recent alcohol consumption

Friedrich Martin Wurst[1]
Joerg Metzger[2]
Katja Jachau[3]
Stephan Seidl[4]
Lutz Pridzun[5]
Ines Janda[6]
Andreas Alt[6]

Psychiatric University Hospital, University of Basel[1], Switzerland
Department of Hydrochemistry and Hydrobiology, University of Stuttgart[2], Germany
Departments of Forensic Medicine, Universities of Magdeburg[3], Erlangen[4] and Ulm[6], Germany
Mediagnost Inc., Reutlingen, Germany

Friedrich Martin Wurst
Psychiatric University Hospital
Wilhelm Klein-Strasse 27
CH – 4025 Basel
Switzerland

Phone: +41-61-325 5112
FAX: +41-61-325 5583
Email: friedrich.wurst@pukbasel.ch

Abstract

In clinical as well as in forensic practice, occupational medicine, at court, for both traffic safety and safety at workplaces biological state markers of high sensitivity and specificity, capable of monitoring those in treatment for alcohol dependence or poly-drug-abusers as well as social drinkers in risky situations (driving, workplaces) are required. The known markers can not be considered to be satisfying with regard to these parameters. Furthermore, they do not cover the whole time axis for alcohol intake - i.e. there is a gap with regard to alcohol consumption of between 1 day and 1 - 2 weeks between short- and long-term-markers like ethanol, methanol, HTOL/HIAA ratio and CDT, GGT or MCV respectively. These traditional markers are in many cases besides alcohol influenced by age, gender and a variety of substances and non-alcohol-associated diseases. Ethyl glucuronide (EtG) is a non-volatile, water-soluble, stable upon storage, direct metabolite of ethanol with a molecular weight of 222 g/mol that can be detected in body fluids, tissues and hair. With its specific time frame of detection intermediate between between short- and long term markers and a high sensitivity and specificity, ethyl glucuronide is a promising marker of alcohol consumption in general that can be detected for an extended time period after the complete elimination of alcohol from the body and a marker for relapse control that enables the therapist to intervene at an early stage of relapsing behaviour.

This review highlights for what purposes and to what extent ethyl glucuronide could be a useful tool to enrich our clinical as well as forensic work. Furthermore the current methods of determination are discussed and future perspectives are given.

Introduction

Both in developing countries and in industrialised societies mental problems account for about 10% of lost healthy years in life. Furthermore 5 of the 10 leading causes of disability world-wide (major depression, schizophrenia, bipolar disorders, alcohol use, obsessive compulsive disorders) are mental problems. In 1990 there have been 288 million cases of alcohol related diseases, which is about 5 times the number of schizophrenia in that year (http://www.who.int/inf-fs/en/fact217.html). Therefore, to monitor alcohol consumption in clinical as well as in forensic practice, occupational medicine, at court and for both traffic safety and safety at workplaces, biological state markers of high sensitivity and specificity capable of monitoring those in treatment for alcohol dependence or poly-drug-abusers as well as social drinkers are required e.g. to improve therapy outcome and quality of life of the patients, increase safety at workplaces and in traffic, avoid harm to the unborn during pregnancy (fetal alcohol syndrome), reduce costs, by making therapy more effective and reduce productivity loss. Among the biological markers which reflect alcohol consumption – usually referred to as "state markers" - major issues restrict their use:

1) the *time spectrum of detection,* they reflect (e.g. only hours for serum ethanol),
2) the *amount of alcohol to be consumed before they are elevated* (e.g. >1000g of ethanol within two weeks for CDT),
3) the *availability and practicability of the test* (e.g. special labs being required for HTOL/HIAA ratio, EtG, dolichol, acet aldehyde etc),
4) they are in many *cases besides alcohol influenced by age, gender and a variety of substances and non-alcohol-associated diseases* (Gilg and Soyka,1997, WHO/ISBRA progress report, 1997).

Ethanol is eliminated to about 90 to 95 % by oxidation, mainly in the liver via alcohol and aldehyde-dehydrogenase, catalase and the microsomal ethanol oxidizing system. The rest is excreted by the kidney (0.5 - 2 %), the lung (1.6 - 6 %) and the skin (max. 0.5 %) (Mallach, 1986). To some possibly still underestimated extent the inducible aerobic gastrointestinal flora contributes to ethanol oxidation in the gastrointestinal tract (Jokelainen et al., 1997). Until recently, the biotransformation of ethanol to ethyl glucuronide received only limited interest in comparison to hepatic and extrahepatic oxidative metabolism.

Although Thierfelder and von Mering found glucuronidation in rabbits for tertiary alcohols in 1885 it was not until 1901 that by Neubauer (Neubauer, 1901) the detoxifying pathway of alcohol elimination via conjugation with activated glucuronic acid (uridine-5′-diphospho-ß-glucuronic acid) was first described. In 1952 EtG was isolated by Kamil et al. as triacetyl methyl ester from the urine of rabbits. The conjugate was determined in human urine by Jaakonmaki et al.in 1967 and in 1973 by Kozu. The findings have been confirmed in 1983 by Besserer and Schmidt. Conjugation of ethanol with activated glucuronic in the presence of membrane bound mitochondial UDP glucuronyl transferase represents with about

0.5 - 1.5 % of total ethanol elimination (Kamil et al., 1952) a minor detoxifying pathway. Neither the indirect proof via an enzymatic approach with bacterial ß-glucuronidase (Russ, 1992) nor by acid hydrolysis (Weinmann, 1995) lead to satisfying results.

Newer aspects

Since 1994 various groups have taken efforts to improve knowledge on this promising new marker. A synopsis is given in table 1.

In 1995 a 5 step synthesis, analytical data and determination of EtG in serum and urine was reported by Schmitt et.al. With a GC/MS method, using EtG as standard substance, they found after acetylation EtG concentrations of between 3 and 130 mg/l in urine samples from 12 drunken drivers. Our group gained better results by using silyl derivatives than acetyl derivatives and t-butyl glucuronide was used as internal standard (Wurst et al., 1995, 1996). With this method we reported of a detection time of up to 75 hours in urine of 23 alcohol withdrawal patients, all initially alcoholised at hospitalisation. In a drinking experiment with an healthy volunteer (60 g of ethanol consumed within 2 hours) no EtG was determined in urine initially, the EtG curve had a phase delay in comparison to the ethanol curve and ETG was detected much longer than ethanol.

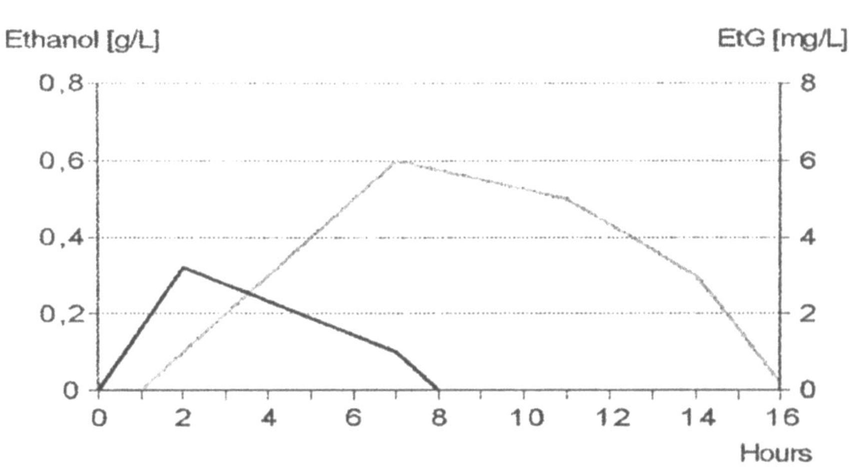

Figure1 Urine ethanol concentration (black) and EtG concentration in urine (grey) are shown from a drinking experiment with an healthy volunteer who consumed 60 g of ethanol within 2 hours. Adapted from :Wurst F. M. et al; Ethylglucuronid - Evaluation eines neuen Alkoholmarkers. In Aktuelle Perspektiven der Biologischen Psychiatrie Möller H.-J., Müller-Spahn F. and Kurtz G. eds. Wien-New York: Springer; 1996: 378-380.

Number and characteristics	Major results	Refrences
23 male alcohol withdrawal patients	UEtG 1 - 100mg/l, detectable up to 80h	*33*
14 drunk drivers	SEC 0.01 - 0.39 %, SEtG 3.2 - 13.7 mg/l UEC 0.01 - 0.20 %, UEtG 3.0 - 130mg/l	*21*
10 male alcohol withdrawal patients 1 volunteer	UEtG 10 - 120 mg/l, detectable up to 84h. phase delay UEC-UEtG, UEC positive for 8 h, UEtG positive for > 14 h	*34*
33 male alcohol withdrawal patients, 181 urine samples d5-EtG as an internal standard	UEC max. 0.40 %, UEtG 3.6 - 710mg/l, detectable up to 75 h	*2*
10 teetotallers 12 healthy volunteers 50 suspected drinking drivers	No ethanol, no EtG detectable SEC max. 0.14 %, SEtG max.3.7mg/l in 13 cases: no SEC, no SEtG detectable in 37 cases: SEtG 0.1 - 20 mg/l	*23*
151 (186) persons undergoing expert assessments for judging driving ability	in 13 (18) cases UEtG 0.1 - 31.9 (45) mg/l	*25, 26*
ELISA 15 serum samples, 22 urine samples	71 % specificity, 100 % sensitivity EtG suggested for „preselection“	*24*
33 alcohol withdrawal patients 30 detoxified patients 43 neurorehabilitating patients	SEC 183mg/dl at hospitalisation UEtG 3.6 - 710 mg/l, detection 57.7+/-16.9h. No correlation with SEC, GGT, MCV, time frame of detection or total amount of clomethiazole required in 4 cases UEtG 4.2 - 196.6 mg/l, in 1 case SEtG 4.8mg/l in 8 urine samples from 7 patients: UEtG 2.9 - 23.49 mg/l	*39*
body fluids and tissues 27 samples from 5 subjects (corpses)	Detection of EtG in gluteal and abdominal fat, liver, brain, serum, urine and CSF	*40*
Spiked serum samples from 1 volunteer and 5 suspected drunk drivers	ESI-LC-MS procedure for serum samples	*15*
9 poly drug abusing patients, 24 alcoholics; 0 days-14weeks hospitalised prior to the study 29 forensic psychiatric inpatients § 64 StGB (penal code) 15 forensic psychiatric inpatients §64 StGB (penal code)	in 4 cases UEtG 0.29 - 1.03 mg/l in 2 cases UEtG 0.3 and 18 mg/l in 1 case UEtG 0.1 mg/l	*43*
14 postmortem hair samples of 4 alcohol misusers, 7 social drinkers and 3 children 10 skin swabs of 2 alcohol misusers, 5 social drinkers and 3 children 6 skin horny layers of 3 social drinkers and 3 children	EtG detectable in hair samples of 2 alcohol misusers and 4 social drinkers EtG detectable in swabs of 2 alcohol misusers and 3 social drinkers EtG detectable in skin samples of 3 social drinkers	*28*
31 hair samples of 16 alcoholics (post-mortem), 4 alcohol withdrawal patients, 6 social drinkers and 5 children	in 14 post-mortem hair samples of alcoholics: 218 – 4025 pg EtG/mg hair, in 4 hair samples of alcohol withdrawal patients:119 – 388 pg EtG/mg; no EtG in hair of social drinkers and children	*4*

(UEtG = urine EtG concentration, UEC = urine ethanol concentration, SEC = serum ethanol concentration, SEtG = serum EtG concentration)

Table 1 Synopsis of major studies on EtG and their results

In 1997(b) Schmitt et al reported on ethyl glucronide concentration in serum of human volunteers, teetotallers and suspected drinking drivers. They found a maximum SEtG of 3.7 mg/l in drinking experiments with up to 90g ethanol, a half life of EtG of 2 - 3 hours and could determine EtG in serum up to 8 hours longer than ethanol. If the SEC is less than 1g/l and SEtG concentration is significantly higher than 5 mg/l, they suggest to assume alcohol misuse.

Deuterium labelled EtG (d_5-EtG) - a gold standard for the determination of EtG because of its with exception of the mass identical physical and chemical parameters - is commercially available since January 1997 (Medichem Inc., Stuttgart, Germany). For the GC/MS procedure after derivatisation with BSTFA Alt et al. from our group performed identification by the mass fragments 160, 261 and 405 and evaluation was by done the ion mass pairs 261/266 and 405/410 (Alt et al., 1997). The detection limit for ethyl glucuronide was 0.1mg/l. With this new tool we found ethyl glucuronide concentrations ranging between 3.6 and 710 mg/l initially and a time frame of detection up to 80 hours when we remeasured the urine samples (stored at -18^0 C) of 33 alcohol withdrawal patients, all alcoholised with a mean BEC of 183 mg/dl at hospitalisation (Wurst et al., 1999a). After detoxification no EtG can be found in urine. For the same patients we found no correlation between the concentration of EtG in urine at hospitalisation and the blood ethanol concentration (BEC) (r=0.17), the time frame of detection (r=0.5) or the total amount of clomethiazole required for the treatment of withdrawal symptoms (r=0.28) (Wurst et al., 1999a). Furthermore we investigated the stability of EtG in urine by measuring the ethanol metabolite in an autosampler at room temperature every hour for 140 h. The results of the internal ratio EtG/d_5EtG fall within a very narrow range. This is of particular interest if the EtG test becomes of widespread use in relation to the stability of samples during storage and transport. EtG also proved its usefulness in the expert assessment for judging driving ability (Seidl et al., 1998). Meanwhile 18 out of 186 cases have been found to be positive for UEtG (Seidl et al., 1999). None of the traditional markers including GGT, MCV or CDT had given an indication for alcohol consumption in these cases.

Ethyl glucuronide in hair samples

Although already in 1994 results of hair analysis of 6 cases were reported by Aderjan et al. and an abstract by Skopp et al from the same group followed in 1995 as well as a further case report in a proceedings by Sachs in 1997, the analysis of this material still is not common and it was not until the year 2000, that systematical experiments with larger sample numbers were performed. In this year, Pragst and colleagues reported to have failed in the analysis of EtG in 3 hair samples of heavy alcoholics. They tried to detect EtG by incubation of hair sample buffer extracts with the enzyme glucuronidase by formation and analysis of ethanol, an attempt, that already earlier failed (Russ, 1992).

In contrast, two other groups were successful in the same year Skopp and colleagues reported about analyses of a total of 14 hair samples (Skopp et al., 2000). Three hair samples from children were EtG negative. Two hair samples from 4 alcohol misusers (50 %) were positive, but below the limit of quantification. At least, 4 samples of a total of 7 samples from social drinkers were positive for EtG. Only in one of all positive cases, a quantification was possible (13.8 ng/mg).

Alt and colleagues published data from analyses of 31 hair samples (Alt et al., 2000). 16 hair samples were taken at autopsy from persons with a known history of alcoholism, basing on police investigations and informations from family practitioners. Four hair samples were taken from alcoholics who were hospitalised for alcohol withdrawal. Six hair samples were from social drinkers with a self reported alcohol consumption of less than 20 g per day. At last, five hair samples came from children who had never consumed alcohol during their life. In 18 out of 31 hair samples analysed, ethyl glucuronide was detected. In 14 of 16 hair samples collected from autopsy cases, EtG concentrations between 218 and 4025 pg/mg hair were measured. In all four hair samples from alcohol withdrawal patients, EtG concentrations between 119 and 388 pg/mg hair were detected. However, measurable concentrations of EtG were not detected in hair from six social drinkers with a self reported daily ethanol consumption of up to 20 g .

ESI-LC/MS-MS and ELISA

For an even more widespread use of ethyl glucuronide as a marker of alcohol consumption a quick and simple method like an ELISA would be of great advantage. Schmitt et al reported in 1998 about an ELISA they had developed together with BIOGENES INC in Berlin. The authors suggested the use of the ELISA for preselection purposes. The results of 37 serum and urine samples however were not quite convincing and until today no further publication or the possibility to obtain this ELISA commercially followed.

Marked methodical improvement and cost reduction was achieved by the development of a LC/MS-MS method with the advantage of no derivatisation being required. Reports on the determination of urine samples (Wurst et al., 1999a,1999c) were shortly followed by the application for serum samples (Nishikawa et al., 1999, Wurst et al., 1999d, Wurst et al., 2000a). For the ESI-LC-MS/MS we used a triple-quadrupole mass spectrometer API 365 (Sciex, Thornhill, Canada) equipped with a nebulizer-assisted electrospray (TurboIonSpray TM) source for detection. Whereas our group like for the GC/MS procedure uses d_5-EtG as internal standard and a double MS, Nishikawa et al. perform the analysis with ethyl glucuronide as standard substance and a single MS. Data were acquired in the MRM (Multiple Reaction Monitoring) mode. Analyte quantification was by peak area ratio. The MS-MS ion transitions monitored were m/z 221 - 75 for EtG and 226 - 75 for d_5-EtG.

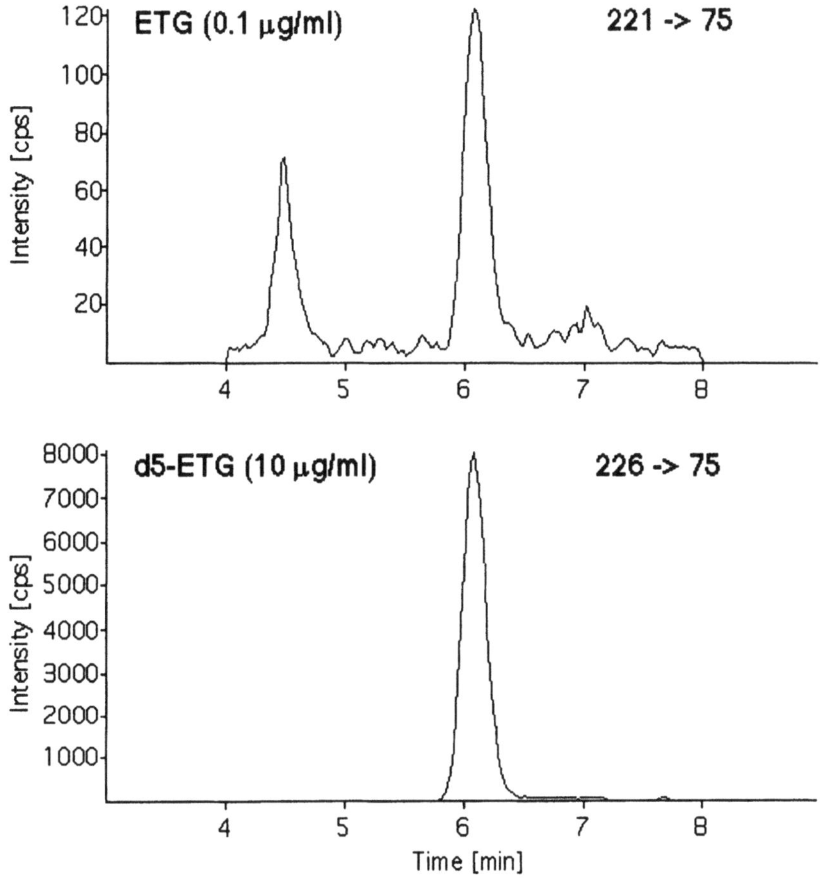

Figure 2 MRM chromatograms of a serum sample. The MS/MS ion transitions shown are 221→ 75 (above) and 226 →75 (below)

Ethyl glucuronide in various body fluids and tissues

We subsequently developed a LC/MS-MS procedure for the analysis of tissue samples to contribute to the question of distribution and storage of EtG in various body fluids and tissues. The purpose of the data on 5 corpses (Wurst et al., 1999d) was to emphasize through our preliminary data the possibility that addition to serum, urine and hair, EtG can also be detected in post-mortem urine, serum, gluteal and abdominal fat, liver, brain and CSF. It remains to be elucidated why

EtG was not found in the liver of one alcoholic and in the gluteal fat of another alcoholic who died with an alcohol intoxication.

Therapeutic use of ethyl glucuronide

EtG also proved its usefulness in general inpatient psychotherapy, were the co-morbidity with substance abuse is well known and known to complicate the treatment as well as in cases of psychotherapy with forensic psychiatric addicted inpatients. The forensic inpatients described were all sentenced according to § 64 StGB (penal code), an option of german law if someone commits a substance-related offence and is deemed to have decreased or no legal responsibility (§20/21 StGB) if at the time of the crime the offender's capability of recognizing the wrongfulness of the action, or to act out of this understanding is considerably impaired. The treatment of these patients is of particular interest to the public as well as to politics and therapists have high responsibility in this special setting. 13 of 20 urine samples from 11 patients of general psychotherapy inpatients were found to be positive for EtG. In more than 200 urine samples from over 100 forensic psychiatric addicted inpatients in different hospitals we found a detection i.e. lapse rate of 5 - 10 % at each a single occasion in cases where neither traditional markers nor the therapist's rating gave an indication for a slip. (Wurst et al., 1999a,c,d). These results underline earlier findings, that ethyl glucuronide is capable of detecting alcohol consumption of patients in cases where neither traditional biological state markers of alcohol intake nor clinical impression gave an indication for relapse. EtG can thus enable the therapist to intervene at an early stage of the lapsing behaviour. Whereas EtG is a useful biological state marker of recent alcohol consumption, preleminary data from our 6 years catamnestic data on 33 patients indicate that EtG probably has no prognostic properties regarding rehospitalisations, seizures etc. (Wurst et al., 2000b).

Discussion

To help closing the gap on the time axis with regard to recent alcohol consumption of between 1 day to 2 weeks between short- and long-term-markers like ethanol, methanol, HTOL/HIAA ratio and CDT, GGT or MCV respectively biological state markers of high sensitivity and specificity capable of monitoring alcohol consumption of those in treatment for alcohol dependence or poly-drug-abusers are required. With its specific time frame of detection intermediate between between short- and long term markers and a high sensitivity and specificity, ethyl glucuronide is a promising marker of alcohol consumption in general that can be detected for an extended time period after the complete elimination of alcohol from the body and a marker for relapse control. With the possibility to detect alcohol consumption up to 70 h after the complete elimination of alcohol from the body EtG covers a unique time spectrum.

The 5-hydroxytryptophol/5-hydroxyindole-3-acetic acid ratio - an other marker that allows the detection of a single relapse - gives a safe proof in cases with values > 15 and up to 15 hours after ethanol elimination only (Helander et al., 1992a,b, 1997). Another promising marker of recent alcohol consumption is methanol. It is discussed that serum methanol concentrations of > 10 mg/l are found after an alcoholisation lasting for at least 10 - 12 hours (Gilg and Soyka, 1997).

As the chemical and physical parameters of d_5-EtG, with exception of the mass, are identical to those of ethyl glucuronide, deuterium-labelled ethyl glucuronide must be considered to be a gold internal standard. The different results of various research groups might be influenced by the following parameters:

1) the *patient groups* per se as well as the *drinking pattern* (Aderjan et al., 1994; Alt et al, 1997, 1999, 2000; Nishikawa et al., 1999; Pragst et al., 2000; Russ, 1992; Sachs,1997; Schmitt et al., 1995, 1997a,b, 1998; Seidl et al., 1998, 1999; Skopp et al., 1995, 2000; Spiegel, 1997; Sticht et al., 1997; Weinmann, 1995; Wurst et al., 1995, 1996a,b, 1997, 1998 a, b, 1999a.d, 2000a,b),
2) using no (Nishikawa et al., 1999; Schmitt et al., 1995, 1997a,b, 1998) or propyl glucuronide (Sticht et al., 1997) as *internal standard* as well as
3) doing an *acetylation* (Nishikawa et al., 1999; Schmitt et al., 1995, 1997a,b, 1998) instead of *silylation* with BSTFA (Alt et al, 1997, 1999, 2000; Seidl et al., 1998, 1999; Wurst et al., 1995, 1996a,b, 1997, 1998 a, b, 1999a.d, 2000a,b) and
4) using a *single MS vs a double MS* (Nishikawa et al., 1999; Wurst et al.,1999a.d, 2000a,b).

As EtG has a longer half life than ethanol an accumulation of EtG must be assumed and was confirmed in our findings as well as elsewhere (Alt et al., 1997, Schmitt et al., 1995, 1997b, Wurst et al., 1999a). No measurable ethyl glucuronide concentrations are observed in serum or urine of non-relapsing patients, non drinking drivers or teetotallers (Alt et al., 1997; Schmitt et al., 1995, 1997a,b; Wurst et al., 1996, 1999a, 1999c, 2000a).

Taking together the results of all subjects tested for EtG up to now we find an additional detection rate of relapses of 5 - 10 % at a single occasion in comparison with the also determined traditional markers like ethanol, CDT, GGT, MCV or the therapist's rating. From our data on more than 1400 urine and serum samples of 183 patients and 186 drivers and the results of other research groups as well as because of theoretical considerations like the fact that EtG is a direct metabolite of ethanol, there is no good reason to contradict the idea of an extraordinary high sensitivity and specificity of ethyl glucuronide as a biological state marker of alcohol consumption.

As EtG is capable of monitoring alcohol consumption of those in treatment for alcohol dependence or poly-drug-abuse, drivers and comorbid alcohol abuse of psychotherapy patients, it can contribute to make treatment more effective and reduce costs. The importance of this new marker is demonstrated not only by an

increasing number of publications and the use of ethyl glucuronide by therapists, forensic toxicologists and judges but also by the fact that our group has been included as assay center in the WHO/ISBRA study on biological state and trait markers of alcohol use and dependence (32). The results from this unique study about to be published and will underline the hypothesis and earlier findings that EtG is an sensitive, specific and reliable marker of recent alcohol intake (Wurst et al., submitted). For further dissemination of tests for EtG availability, practicability and further reduction of test costs will be crucial. GC/MS and more and more also LC/MS-MS are available almost ubiquitary. Hair analysis and the development of an ELISA are future perspectives. As however EtG is a rather small molecule with a molecular weight of 222 g/mol, this is a difficulty with regard to creating an antibody. However, a first immunization of 2 BALB/c mice with a mixture of an EtG-KLH conjugate with one lipopeptide conjugate - first fusion (after 7 weeks) of the spleen of one immunized mouse - gave one positive, a second fusion (after 15 weeks) of mouse 2 gave 10 positive clones.
Like in the monitoring of illicit drugs, the determination of the specific weight or the creatinine value of urine can contribute to exclude manipulation of the samples. Studies regarding the glucuronidation and ß-glucuronidase activity are required to elucidate interindividual, intraindividual and dose dependent differences in formation and degradation of EtG and are an ongoing activity of our group.
The complementary use of this marker with a specific time frame of detection with other biological state markers like fatty acid ethyl esters, HTOL/HIAA ratio and phosphatidyl ethanol should lead via the possibility of therapeutic intervention at early stages of lapsing behaviour to significant improvement in treatment outcome, therapy effectiveness and cost reduction.

References

Aderjan R., Besserer H., Sachs H., Schmitt G., Skopp G.; Ethyl glucuronide – a non volatile metabolite in human hair. Lecture on the TIAFT-SOFT Joint Meeting, Tampa 1994.

Alt A., Wurst F. M.; Seidl S.; Bestimmung von Ethylglucuronid in Urinproben mit dem internen Standard d5-Ethylglucuronid. Blutalkohol 34: 360-365; 1997.

Alt A., Kempter Ch., Wurst F. M.; Nachweis und quantitative Bestimmung von Ethyl-glucuronid in Urinproben mittels GC/MS und ESI-LC-MS-MS. Symposiumsband des XI. GTFCH Symposium Mosbach 22. - 24.04. 1999, Verlag Dr. Dieter Helm, Heppenheim, in Druck.

Alt A., Janda, I., Seidl, S., Wurst, F. M.; Determination of ethyl glucuronide in hair samples. Alcohol 35: 313-314; 2000.

Besserer K., Schmidt V.; Ein Beitrag zur renalen Ausscheidung von Äthylglucuronid nach oraler Alkoholaufnahme. Zentralblatt Rechtsmedizin 25: 369; 1983.

Gilg Th., Soyka M.; Wertigkeit biologischer Marker für Alkoholabusus und Alkoholismus. Nervenheilkunde 16: 362-371;1997.

Helander A., Beck O., Jacobsson G., Wikström T., Borg S.; Characterization of elevated urinary 5-hydroxytryptophol as a marker of recent alcohol consumption. Alcoholism: Clin Exp Res 16: 607; 1992.

Helander A., Wikström T., Löwenmo C., Jacobsson G., Beck O.; Urinary excretion of 5-hydroxyindole-3-acetic acid and 5-hydroxytryptophol after oral loading with serotonine. Life Sci 50: 1207-1213; 1992.

Helander A., Beck O., Borg S.; 5-Hydroxytryptophol (5HTOL), a new sensitive urinary test of recent alcohol consumption. In Proceedings of the 14th International Conference on Alcohol, Drugs and Traffic Safety, Annecy 1997, Mercier-Guyon, C ed; 1997: 223-228.

Jaakonmaki P. I., Knox K. L., Horning E. C., Horning M. G.; The characterization by gas-liquid chromatography of ethyl-ß-D-glucosiduronic-acid as a metabolite of ethanol in rat and man. Eur J Pharmacol 1: 63-70; 1967.

Jokelainen K., Nosova T., Väkeväinen S., Tilonen J., Salaspuro M.; Bacteriocolonic pathway for ethanol oxidation; Characteristics and induction during chronic alcohol consumption. Alcohol Alcoholism 32: 342; 1997.

Kamil I. A., Smith J. N., Williams R. T.; A new aspect of ethanol metabolism: isolation of ethyl-glucuronide. Biochemical Journal 51: 32-33; 1952.

Kozu T.; Gas chromatographic analysis of ethyl-ß-D-glucuronide in human urine. Shinzu Igaku Zasshi 21: 595-601; 1973.

Mallach H. J.; Konzentrationsverlauf im Blut: Pharmakokinetik. In Alkoholwirkung beim Menschen Mallach H. J, Hartmann H. and Schmidt V. Hrsg; Stuttgart-New York: Thieme Verlag, Stuttgart-New York; 1986: 13-34.

Nishikawa M., Tsuchihashi H., Miki A., Katagi M., Schmitt G., Zimmer H., Keller Th., Aderjan R.; Determination of ethylglucuronide, a minor metabolite of ethanol, in human serum by liquid chromatography-electrospray ionization mass spectrometry. spectrometry J Chromatogr B 726: 105-110; 1999

Neubauer O.; Ueber Glucuronsäurepaarung bei Stoffen der Fettreihe. Arch exp Path Pharmak 46: 133-154; 1901.

Pragst F., Spiegel K, Sporkert F., Bohnenkamp M.; Are there possibilities for the detection of chronically elevated alcohol consumption by hair analysis? A report about the state of investigation. For Sci Int ; 107: 201-223; 2000.

Roine R., Salaspuro M.; Marker für Alkoholismus und alkoholassoziierte Organschäden. In Handbuch Alkohol, Alkoholismus, Alkoholbedingte Organschäden. Seitz H. K., Lieber Ch. S., Simanowski U. A. Hrsg. Johann Ambrosius Barth, Leipzig-Heidelberg, 1995: 93-120.

Russ A.; Ethylglucuronidausscheidung beim Menschen nach länger zurückliegendem Ethanolkonsum. Disertation zur Erlangnung des Doktorgrades der Medizin der Medizinischen Fakultät der Eberhard-Karls-Universität Tübingen, 1992.

Sachs H.; Drogennachweis in Haaren. In Das Haar als Spur - Spuren in Haaren Kijewski H., Hrsg. Reasearch in Legal Medicine, Volume 16. Lübeck: Schmidt-Römhild; 1997: 119-135.

Schmitt G., Aderjan R., Keller Th., Wu M.; Ethyl-Glucuronide: An unusual ethanol metabolite in humans. Synthesis, analytical data, and determination in serum and urine. J Anal Toxicol 19: 91-94; 1995.

Schmitt G., Drönner P., Aderjan R., Skopp G.; Blutprobe mit 1,44 ‰ Ethanol enthielt kein Ethylglucuronid - Fallbericht. Blutalkohol 34: 371-378; 1997a.

Schmitt G., Droenner P., Skopp G., Aderjan R.; Ethyl glucuronide concentrations in serum of human volunteers, teetotalers, and suspected drinking drivers. J Forensic Sci 42: 1099-1102; 1997b.

Schmitt G., Aderjan R. E., Kirchner M., Zimmer H.; Enzymimmunoassy und GC/MS zur Bestimmung von Ethylglucuronid in Serum und Urin. Blutalkohol 35: 428-33; 1998.

Seidl S., Wurst F. M., Alt A.; Überprüfung einer Abstinenzbehauptung in der Fahreignungs-Oberbegutachtung mit Hilfe des Ethanolmetaboliten Ethylglucuronid (EtG). Blutalkohol 35: 174-182; 1998.

Seidl S., Wurst F. M., Alt A.; Der Einsatz des Ethanolmetaboliten Ethylglucuronid in der Fahreignungs-Oberbegutachtung. Tagungsband der 30. Jahrestagung der Deutschen Gesellschaft für Verkehrsmedizin e.V. 10.13.03.1999, Berlin. Berichte der Bundesanstalt für Strassenwesen, in Druck.

Skopp G., Schmitt G., Drönner P., Aderjan R.; Trinkverhalten und Haaranalyse. T+K 62(1):46, 1995.

Skopp G., Schmitt G., Pötsch L., Drönner P., Aderjan R., Mattern R.; Ethyl glucuronide in human hair. Alcohol 2000; 35: 283-285.

Spiegel K.; Untersuchungen zum Nachweis alkoholspezifisch metabolisierter Substanzen aus menschlichen Haaren mit Gaschromatographie-Massenspektrometrie. T+K 64(2): 58-62, 1997.

Sticht G., Käferstein H., Staak M.; GC-MS-Bestimmung von Ethylglucuronid im Serum mit Propylglucuronid als internem Standard. Rechtsmedizin 7: 184-188; 1997.

Weinmann W. F.; Ethylglucuronid-Ausscheidung beim Menschen während der Resorptions- und frühen Postresorptionsphase nach Alkoholaufnahme. Dissertation zur Erlangnung des Doktorgrades der Medizin der Medizinischen Fakultät der Eberhard-Karls-Universität Tübingen, 1995.

WHO/ISBRA study on biological state and trait markers of alcohol use and dependence: progress report. WHO/MSA/PSA/97.11:1-40; 1997.

Wurst F. M., Seidl S., Sachs H., Besserer K., Hirsch M., Reinhardt G., Schüttler R.; Ethyl glucuronide - Evaluation of a new marker of alcoholism. Alcohol and Alcoholism 30: 560; 1995.

Wurst F. M., Seidl S., Sachs H., Besserer K., Reinhardt G., Schüttler R.; Ethylglucuronid - Evaluation eines neuen Alkoholmarkers. Vortrag bei der 6.Jahrestagung der „Deutschen Gesellschaft für Biologische Psychiatrie" in München, Okt.1994. In Aktuelle Perspektiven der Biologischen Psychiatrie Möller H.-J., Müller-Spahn F. and Kurtz G. Hrsg. Wien-New York: Springer; 1996: 378-380.

Wurst F. M., Seidl S., Sachs H., Gilg T., Hirsch M., Reinhardt G., Schüttler R.; Ethyl glucuronide - Evaluation of a new marker of alcoholism and comparison to traditional alcohol markers. J Neurol 243: 24-25; 1996.

Wurst F. M., Seidl S., Alt A.; Ethyl glucuronide - evaluation of a new marker of alcoholism by deutericed standard. Alcohol Alcoholism 32: 327; 1997.

Wurst F. M., Seidl S., Alt A.; Ethylglukuronid - Evaluation eines Single relapse markers. Nervenarzt 69: 84; 1998a.

Wurst F. M., Seidl S., Alt A.; Ethyl glucuronide - a metabolite of alcohol with clinical and forensic implications. Alcoholism : Clin Exp Res 22/3 Suppl.:140A.; 1998b.

Wurst F. M., Kempter Ch., Seidl S., Alt A.; Ethyl glucuronide - a marker of alcohol consumption and a relapse marker with clinical and forensic implications. Alcohol Alcoholism 34: 71-77; 1999a.

Wurst F. M., Schüttler R., Kempter Ch., Seidl S., Gilg Th., Jachau K., Alt A.; Can ethyl glucuronide be determined in postmortem body fluids and tissues? Alcohol Alcoholism 34/ 2: 260-261; 1999b.

Wurst F. M., Kempter Ch., Metzger J., Seidl S., Alt A.; Der Ethanolmetabolit Ethylglucuronid - ein Marker für Alkoholkonsum. Psycho 25: 42-45; 1999c.

Wurst F. M., Seidl S., Jachau K., Kempter Ch., Alt A.; Ethyl glucuronide - Determination of a marker of recent alcohol consumption with clinical and forensic implications in various body fluids and tissues. Alcohol Alcoholism 34/3: 446; 1999d.

Wurst F. M., Kempter Ch., Metzger J., Seidl S., Alt A.; Ethyl glucuronide - a marker of recent alcohol consumption with clinical and forensic implications. Alcohol 20: 111-116; 2000.

Wurst F. M., Janda I., Metzger J., Seidl S., Alt A.; Ethyl glucuronide – new aspects of the marker of alcohol consumption. Alcoholism: Clin Exp Res 24/5 Suppl.:140A.; 2000.

Wurst F.M., Metzger J. and the WHO/ISBRA study on biological state and trait markers of alcohol use and dependence. The direct ethanol metabolite ethyl glucuronide is a specific marker of recent alcohol consumption. Alcoholism: Clin Exp Res (submitted)

Phosphatidylethanol; clinical significance and biochemical basis

Arthur Varga
Kristian Moller
Per Hansson
Steina Aradottir
Christer Alling

Department of Medical Neurochemistry
Institute of Laboratory Medicine
Lund University Hospital
SE-221 85 Lund
Sweden

1. Biology of PEth
2. Analysis of PEth
3. PEth as a marker of alcohol abuse
4. Conclusions

Acknowledgements

This project was supported by grants from Trygg Hansa, the Swedish Medical Research Council, Systembolagets Fond för Alkoholforskning, and Direktör Albert Påhlssons Stiftelse för Forskning och Välgörenhet.

1. Biology of Phosphatidylethanol (PEth)

Ethanol metabolism

As shown in figure 1, ethanol can be metabolized by oxidative and nonoxidative pathways (Lieber, 1995). In the oxidative pathway, ethanol is converted to acetaldehyde through the action of alcohol dehydrogenases, the microsomal ethanol-oxidizing system, or catalase. Acetaldehyde is then subsequently metabolized to acetate through the action of aldehyde dehydrogenases. In one of the nonoxidative pathways of ethanol metabolism, ethanol undergoes esterification with fatty acids by the action of fatty acid ethyl ester synthase to form fatty acid ethyl esters. The nonoxidative ethanol pathway that is the focus of this review is the pathway leading to the synthesis of phosphatidylethanol. Figure 1 shows how ethanol can be inserted as the head group of a phospholipid to form phosphatidylethanol. The transformation occurs through the activation of phospholipase D, mainly on phosphatidylcholine in the presence of ethanol.

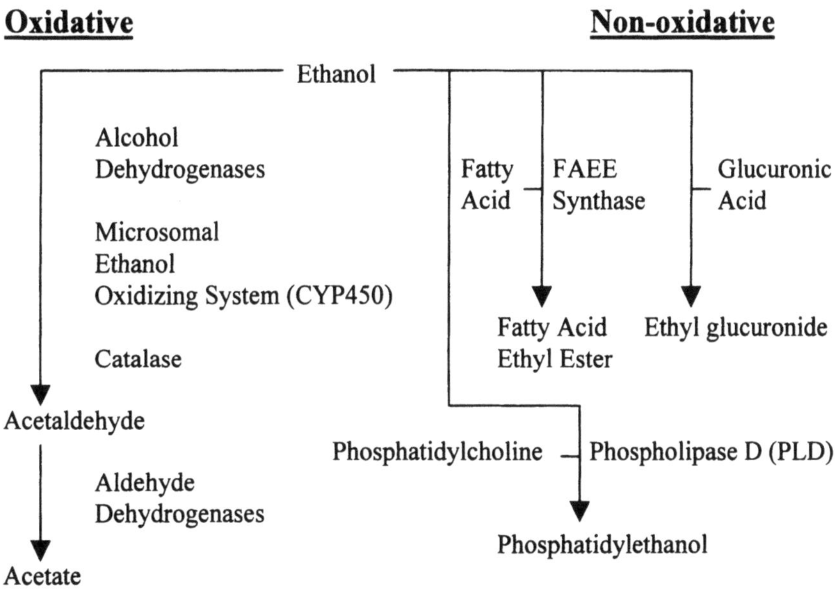

Figure 1 Oxidative and nonoxidative pathways of ethanol metabolism

Formation of PEth

Phosphatidylethanol (PEth) is an abnormal phospholipid, which is formed in cell membranes only in the presence of ethanol (Alling et al., 1983). The formation of PEth in mammalian cells is catalysed by PLD (Gustavsson & Alling, 1987; Kobayashi & Kanfer, 1987). Since PEth is formed instead of phosphatidic acid in the presence of ethanol, a reduction of phosphatidic acid production will occur. The inhibitory effect on phosphatidic acid formation is dependent on the ethanol concentration (Konishi et al., 1991; Mizunuma et al., 1993; Gustavsson & Hansson, 1990; Pai et al., 1987), but can also differ between different cells and tissues at given ethanol concentrations (Horwitz, 1991; Gruchalla et al., 1990; Kanaho et al., 1991; Lin et al., 1991) Since PEth is a phospholipid which does not normally occur, it may affect cell function and therefore be responsible for some of the effects of ethanol on cells. The amount of PEth formed is crucial for the possible effects. Intraperitoneal injection of ethanol to rats produced the highest levels of PEth in forebrain and kidney (12 - 28 nmol/g wet weight) 1 - 2 h after the injection and corresponded to about 0.02 - 0.05 % of the total phospholipids (Gatalica et al., 1993; Lundqvist et al., 1994b). After one week of ethanol exposure of rats, there was a higher amount of PEth in forebrain (28 nmol/g ww) compared to that formed after a single injection (12 nmol/g ww), despite a lower blood alcohol concentration due to metabolic tolerance (Lundqvist et al., 1994b) This indicates that a further accumulation of PEth seems to occur after chronic exposure to ethanol via repeated intraperitoneal injections.

Degradation of PEth

The degradation rate is also of major importance for the amount accumulating. In cells and tissues so far studied, the degradation of PEth is relatively slow (Gustavsson, 1995). In intact pancreatic islets about 50 % of endogenously formed PEth remained after 2 h of incubation (Metz & Dunlop, 1990). In NG108-15 cells in which exogenously added PEth had been incorporated into the membrane a 31 - 46 % decrease was observed after 60 min (Lundqvist et al., 1993) and when the mass of endogenously formed PEth was analyzed in intact rat hepatocytes a 40 % decrease was seen after 60 min (Moehren et al., 1994). In rat Leydig cells, the degradation of endogenously formed PEth was slightly faster; a 59 % decrease after 60 min (Vinggard & Hansen, 1993). In rat brain, the T½ of PEth was 8 - 10 h and detectable levels were observed up to 20 h after a single intraperitoneal injection of 3 g of ethanol/kg of body weight (Lundqvist et al., 1994b). In neutrophils from chronic alcoholics, PEth was detected as long as 23 h after the last ethanol intake (Lundqvist et al., 1994a). Analysis of detectable PEth in whole blood from alcoholics, was possible up to 3 weeks after the last ethanol intake (Gunnarsson et al., 1998), which is considerably longer than has been observed previously in any other tissue or cell. The mechanism for PEth degradation has not been elucidated. Although isolated phospholipase A2 (Pai et al., 1987) and PLD (Alling et al., 1984) will degrade PEth in vitro, there is no report so far about the kind of phospholipases that are involved in the degradation of PEth in vivo.

Molecular species of PEth

The fatty acid composition of PEth may be important for its effects on cell function and perhaps also for degradation of PEth. PEth formed in organs from ethanol-treated rats has been studied. Brain PEth contained high proportions of palmitic and oleic acids. Lower proportions of the polyunsaturated fatty acids arachidonic acids and docosahexanoic acids, were also found (Alling et al., 1984). In liver, on the other hand, palmitic, stearic and arachidonic acids were the dominating fatty acids of PEth (Alling et al., 1984). These fatty acid compositions were not identical to any other phospholipid. PEth formed after agonist stimulation has however showed fatty acid compositions, similar to other phospholipids. Bradykinin or phorbol ester stimulation of PC12 cells (Holbrook et al., 1992) and phorbol ester stimulation of NG108-15 (Boyano-Adánez et al., 1994) both produced PEth with fatty acids similar to those found in phosphatidylcholine. Noradrenaline- and ionomycin-stimulated as well as basal phospholipase D activity from rat hippocampus produced two different classes of PEth from two different classes of phosphatidylcholine, enriched with arachidonic acid and myristic acid respectively (Sarri et al., 1996). It was suggested that two molecular classes of phosphatidylcholine may be the main substrates for PLD in rat hippocampus. In relation to fatty acid composition, PEth species with acyl-, alkyl, as well as alkenyl-linked chains have been demonstrated (Hii et al., 1989; Daniel et al., 1993; Tou et al., 1999).

Biophysical effects of PEth on membranes and membrane enzymes

PEth is a negatively charged phospholipid with a small , hydrophobic head group. Compared both with the precursor phospholipids, phosphatidylcholine, phosphatidyl ethanolamine and phosphatidylinositol, and the normal product of PLD activity, phosphatidic acid, it differs in both head group size and charge. PEth, being hydrophobic, may disrupt the membrane surface interlipid lattice of electrostatic interactions and hydrogen bonds (Browning, 1981; Omodeo-Salé et al., 1989). PEth increases the fluidity in both phosphatidylcholine vesicles and a crude brain membrane fraction. Notably, PEth-containing membranes are partly resistant to the fluidizing effect of ethanol (Omodeo-Salé et al., 1991). However, a higher concentration of PEth is required for the effects on natural membrane preparations compared with the changes induced in phosphatidylcholine vesicles. It has been shown that PEth confers tolerance to the ethanol-induced membrane disordering effect in lipid vesicles containing phosphatidylcholine and phosphatidylethanolamine (Rottenberg et al., 1992). Bondeson and Sundler (1987) studied the susceptibility of PEth-containing vesicles towards Ca2+-induced fusion. Phosphatidylethanol-rich vesicles were relatively resistant to Ca2+-induced fusion, but were highly sensitive to proton-induced fusion. The transbilayer distribution of PEth has been studied in unilamellar vesicles, mixed with phosphatidylcholine (Victorov et al., 1994). In both large and small vesicles, PEth preferred the inner leaflet. Interestingly, PEth was rapidly redistributed to the outer leaflet after addition of millimolar concentrations of Ca2+ and other multivalent cations. This is another property of PEth that is different from other lipids. Phosphatidylethanol may affect membrane-associated enzymes. In crude brain membrane fraction, the Vmax of Na+-K+-ATPase was decreased by PEth (Omodeo-Salé et al., 1991). Ethanol (5 - 50 mM) induced an increase in the Na+-K+-ATPase activity but this increase was only 20 % in membranes containing PEth. The membrane-associated enzyme, 5'-nucleotidase, was also affected by ethanol, showing an increase in Vmax in the presence of PEth (Omodeo-Salé et al., 1991). PEth has also been shown to stimulate the plasma-membrane Ca2+-pump from human erythrocytes (Suju et al., 1996).

Effects of PEth on signal transduction

Effects of PEth on cell signalling processes have been studied. In a study on NG108-15 cells containing exogenously synthesized PEth, basal levels of the second messenger, inositoltrisphosphate (IP3), were increased (Lundqvist et al., 1993). The same effect was also observed with endogenously formed PEth in the cells, after treatment with 100 mM ethanol for 2 days (Lundqvist et al., 1993). Other findings indicate that PEth added in vitro to rat cerebellar membranes reduces the binding of IP3 to the IP3 receptors (Rodríguez et al., 1994). Chronic ethanol treatment of rats was also found to reduce the IP3 binding (Rodríguez et al., 1994; Rodríguez et al., 1996). Effects of PEth on PKC have also been described (Asaoka et al., 1988). In vitro, PEth could replace phosphatidylserine in activating PKC and the effect was most effective for the brain-specific γ-isoform of the enzyme, compared to the α- and β-forms (Asaoka et al., 1988). In another study, PEth was demonstrated to decrease the phosphatidylserine requirement of PKCα, PKCβ and PKCγ in a mixed micelle system (Lee and Bell, 1992). Of the effects on transmitter release, a report showed reduced release of noradrenaline altered by PEth in SH-SY5Y cells (Purkiss, 1994).

Phospholipase D (PLD)

PLD-induced hydrolysis of PC in the plasma membrane triggers the formation of the anionic lipid phosphatidic acid (PA) and the polar head group choline (Exton 1997, Exton 1998). PA is an important second messenger (Billah 1993, Exton 1994) whereas choline constitutes a precursor for the synthesis of the neurotransmitter acetylcholine. Most cellular effects elicited by PLD are mediated by PA, including modulation of protein tyrosine phosphatase activity (Tomic et al. 1995), increased actin "stress fiber" formation (Cross et al. 1996), organelle translocation and endocytosis (Liscovitch et al. 2000) and mitosis (Boarder 1994, Kötter and Klein 1999). PA can be dephosphorylated into the potent PKC-activator 1,2-diacylglycerol (DAG) by phosphatidate phosphohydrolases (PPHs) (Brindley and Waggoner 1998) and/or into lysophosphatidic acid (lyso-PA) by a specific PLA2 (Moolenaar 1995). DAG is reconverted into PA by DAG kinases (Topham and Prescott 1998).

Mammalian PLD subtypes

The molecular cloning of PLD-members from a wide range of prokaryotic and eukaryotic organisms (Morris et al. 1996) has revealed a unique and evolutionarily well conserved gene superfamily (Hammond et al. 1995) with insignificant homology to other known phospholipases, including PLC (Exton 1997).

The cDNAs for two mammalian PLD-subtypes (PLD1 and PLD2) were recently cloned. PLD1 has been cloned from human (Hammond et al. 1995, Steed et al. 1998), mouse (Colley et al. 1997a) and rat (Park et al. 1997). Additionally, two alternative splice-forms of PLD1 (PLD1a and PLD1b) occur in rat and human (Hammond et al. 1997, Park et al. 1997, Steed et al., 1998). The shorter form, PLD1b lacking 38 amino acids at corresponding regions in the rat and human PLD1, is similar to PLD1a in catalytic activity. PLD2 is 52% identical with PLD1 at the nucleotide level and has been cloned from mouse (Colley et al. 1997b), rat

(Kodaki and Yamashita 1997) and man (Lopez et al. 1998, Steed et al. 1998). Apart from the full-length form of human PLD2, additional truncated variants of human PLD2 have been cloned (Steed et al. 1998). Pedersen et al. (1998) have cloned a third mammalian supergene family member, Sam-9 from a mouse brain cDNA library. This protein shows structural features reminiscent of other PLD supergene family members, although it remains unknown whether Sam-9 displays PLD-like catalytic activity.

PLD-activity in mammalian cells

Mammalian PLD was originally isolated from brain membrane fractions (Kanfer 1980) and was found to be activated by oleate with a preference for PC as substrate.

Two biochemically distinct forms of PC-specific PLD have been identified; those that can be stimulated by unsaturated fatty acids (oleate) and those that are activated by ADP-ribosylating factor (ARF), a small GTPase-binding protein (Cockcroft 1997, Frohman et al. 1999).

It is known that PLD1 is involved in the regulation of intracellular secretion and intracellular membrane trafficking (Roth et al. 1999). The main function of PLD2 seems to be related to activity-dependent remodelling of the actin cytoskeleton and endocytotic processes (Colley et al. 1997b).

Regulation of PLD-activity

The activity of PLD1 and PLD2 is dependent upon phosphatidyl inositol 4-,5-bisphosphate (PIP2) (Liscovitch et al. 1994, Sciorra et al. 1999). PLD1 displays a very low basal activity and requires complexing with cytosolic factors to become fully active. These factors, which act in synergy, include PKCα- and -β (Kiss 1996, Cockcroft 1997, Frohman et al. 1999, Zhang et al. 1999), the small GTPase-binding proteins, cdc42 (Han et al. 1998), Ral (Luo et al. 1998), RhoA (Hammond et al. 1995, Cockcroft 1997, Frohman et al. 1999) and the ARFs (Brown and Sternweis 1995, Cockcroft 1997, Frohman et al. 1999). Although PLD2 is constitutively active in vivo, (Kodaki and Yamashita 1997) the catalytic activity of this PLD-subtype is sligthly elevated by ARF (Sung et al. 1999).

PLD-activity can be stimulated by various ligands (Meier et al. 1999) including neurotransmitters, regulatory peptides and extracellular signaling molecules that couple to the activation of tyrosine kinase receptors (Zhang et al. 1992, Slaaby et al. 1998) and G-protein-coupled receptors (Boyano-Adánez et al. 1997, Mitchell et al. 1998, Albani-Torregrossa et al. 1999).

Localization of PLD

The PLD subtypes differ in their pattern of intracellular and intercellular localization (Meier et al. 1999). PLD1 is subcellularly localized to perinuclear compartments (Golgi and ER) (Czarny et al. 2000) as well as lysosomes and secretory granules (Brown et al. 1998). Upon cellular stimulation, PLD1 translocates to the plasma membrane (Brown et al. 1998). PLD2, on the other hand is localized to low-density membrane microdomains together with caveolae in the plasma mem-

brane (Colley et al. 1997b, Czarny et al. 2000) but associates with endosomes upon activation (Colley et al. 1997b).
In the mouse, the highest expression of PLD1 mRNA is found in the lung and kidney whereas PLD2 mRNA was most strongly expressed in the brain and lung as analyzed by Northern Blot (Colley et al. 1997a).

Functional domains of the PLD molecule

Analyses of the mammalian PLD-isoforms has revealed molecular consensus domains including two motifs containing well-conserved histidine, lysine, aspartic acid and/or asparagine residues, the "HKD"-motif, forming the active catalytic site (Sung et al. 1999, Frohman et al. 1999, Liscovitch et al. 2000). Computerized database searches in order to identify domains conserved between PLD1 and PLD2 has led to the identification of pleckstrin-homology (PH)-domains (Steed et al. 1998) and transphosphatidylation "signatures" (Steed et al. 1998).

Transphosphatidylation reaction of PLD

Ethanol as well as other primary alcohols, up to 1-octanol (Seidler et al., 1996), acts as co-substrates in the transphosphatidylation reaction of PLD, and substitutes for water in the normal hydrolysis reaction, which results in the corresponding phosphatidyl-alcohol instead of phosphatidic acid (Yu et al., 1996; Liscovitch et al., 1999). This phenomenon was first observed in plants (Dawson, 1967; Yang et al., 1967) but has also been demonstrated in mammalian tissues (Gustavsson and Alling, 1987; Kobayashi and Kanfer, 1987). In addition to the membrane-associated PLD activity, PEth formation has also been demonstrated to be catalysed by the cytosolic form of PLD (Wang et al., 1991). Activation of several different receptor complexes results in increased PLD activity in a variety of cell types, and thereby in PEth formation when ethanol is present (for review, see Billah and Anthes, 1990; Shukla and Halenda, 1991; Thompson et al., 1993; Exton, 1994). PLD has emerged as a widely distributed component of signal transduction cascades. PEth formation, which is only catalysed by PLD, unequivocally indicates the involvement of PLD in signal transduction cascades.

2. Analysis of PEth

Until now, PEth has been measured with mass spectrometry (MS), thin-layer chromatography (TLC) and high pressure liquid chromatography (HPLC). MS offers very definite and accurate measurements of PEth, with detection down to femtomolar levels and knowledge about molecular species (Gunnarsson et al., 1998). MS does however require relatively expensive instrumentation and technical expertice, which might limit its use. Although PEth has been measured with TLC (Hansson et al., 1997), this method is time-consuming and has a relatively high coefficient of variation.
The set-up with HPLC combined with an evaporative light-scattering detector (ELSD) offers a relatively simple and quite accurate way of analyzing PEth.

PEth is measured in whole blood by performing lipid extraction of heparinized blood in organic solvent (hexane:isopropanol 60/40) followed by concentration of sample before analysis with HPLC. The HPLC-ELSD system operates with an autosampler where samples are kept at +4°C until injection. Separation takes place in a heated (55°C) DIOL-type column, where PEth is separated from other lipids by elution with a tertiary gradient. Detection of PEth occurs with an ELSD detector in which the mobile phase is evaporated at 80°C, leaving very small droplets containing PEth. These droplets are hit by laser light which is scattered depending on the amount of molecule in droplets. The light-scattering generates an electrical signal which leads to a computerized data evaluation system. A chromatogram of an analysis is shown in figure 2.

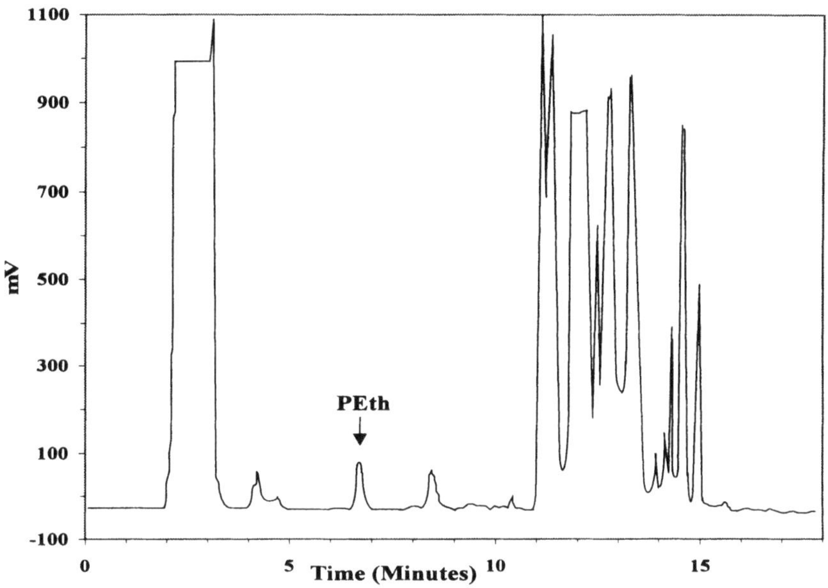

Figure 2 Chromatogram of an HPLC analysis of whole blood extract containing 5 nmol of phosphatidylethanol (PEth). PEth elutes at t=6.7 minutes.

Sensitivity and specificity

The method manages to detect PEth down to 0.2 nmol, equaling 0.8 μmol/liter whole blood. From a study with repeated intake of ethanol it was concluded that a prolonged daily intake of about 50 g ethanol for 3 weeks was enough to raise PEth to detectable levels. (Varga et al., 1998). Because PEth is considered to be formed only as a consequence of ethanol intake (Gustavsson, 1995), the biological specificity should be close to 100 %.

Analytical interference

Interference of ten different drugs commonly used by alcoholics have been investigated. The investigated drugs (citalopram, diazepam, phenytoin, fluoxetine,

carbamazepine, clonazepam, nitrazepam, oxazepam, paroxetine, valproic acid) had a very limited interference on analytical performance (Varga et al., 1998), and further improvements of the method have eliminated any interference of these drugs.
So far no evidence of interfering endogenous substances have been reported, but such substances may occur (e.g. in patients having lipid disorders) and needs to be further investigated.

3. PEth as a Marker of Alcohol Abuse

Level and dose-response of PEth in humans

Recent studies have suggested and given support to use PEth in blood as a marker of alcohol abuse. Chronic alcoholics admitted for detoxification had PEth levels of 13.2 µmol/liter as mean on the first day after admission and remained detectable up to 14 days after admission (Hansson et al., 1997). PEth has been determined in extracts of blood from alcoholics using HPLC-ELSD and electrospray mass spectrometric detection (Gunnarsson et al., 1998). These patients had PEth levels of 5 – 13 µmol/liter and were detectable up to three weeks after the beginning of an alcohol-free period. The molecular species of PEth were found to be similar to those of phosphatidylcholine in one of the patients. A third study on chronic alcoholics showed PEth levels of 2.5 and 5.1 µmol/liter as mean in two different groups respectively (Varga et al., 2000).
A study on healthy volunteers revealed that a single dose of ethanol (32 - 47 g) does not produce measurable amounts of PEth (Varga et al., 1998). However, out of twelve volunteers who had consumed between 624 and 2134 g of ethanol during three weeks, eight persons had detectable levels of PEth (1.0 - 2.1 µmol/liter) (Figure 3). As can be seen in figure 3, a break point of total ethanol intake yielding detectable PEth seems to be around 1000 g, with a mean daily intake of about 50 g. However, more studies have to be performed in order to establish the amount of ethanol and drinking patterns that are required to produce PEth concentrations that exceed the detection limit. Figure 4 summarizes the observed levels of PEth in blood from healthy volunteers with a single-dose and with repeated intake, and PEth in chronic alcoholics.

Blood compartmentalization of PEth

So far analysis of PEth has been performed by using whole blood. It has however been of interest to know if PEth might be unevenly distributed in blood and perhaps be localized in particular cell types. A recent study on blood from chronic alcoholics showed that almost all PEth was found in the erythrocyte fraction (Varga et al., 2000).

Normalization and elimination kinetics of PEth in blood

Previous studies have shown that PEth in blood from alcoholics can be detected up to as long as 3 weeks from the end of a drinking period (Hansson et al., 1997 and Gunnarsson et al., 1998). In a recent study 8 of 15 chronic alcoholics had

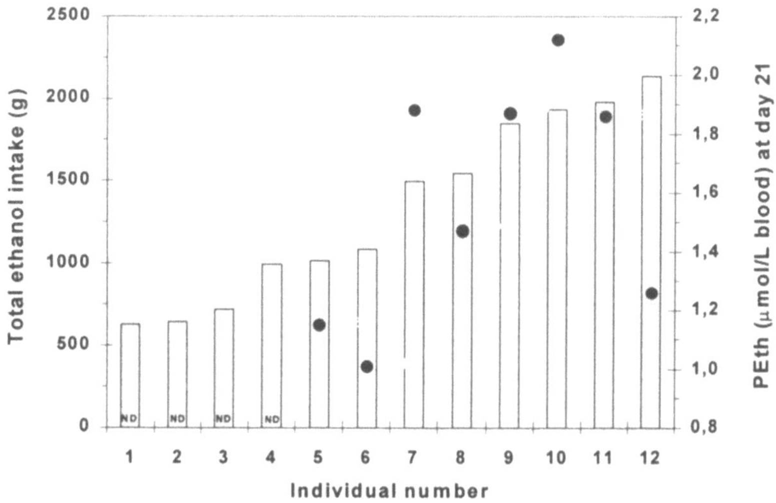

Figure 3 Relationship between estimated total ethanol intake for 3 weeks (staples; grams of pure ethanol), and levels of blood phosphatidylethanol (PEth, represented by dots; µmol/liter whole blood) in 12 healthy volunteers with repeated intake. ND = Not Detectable.

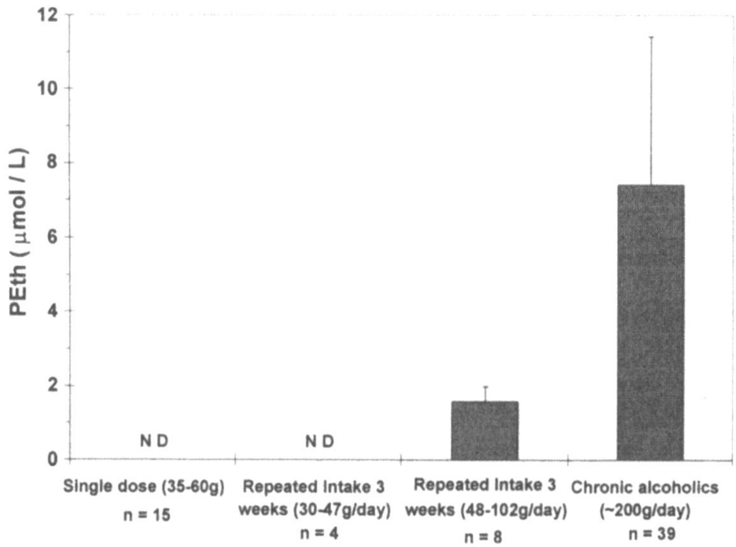

Figure 4 Levels of in vivo phosphatidylethanol (PEth) concentrations found in 4 groups of human subjects with different intakes of ethanol. X-axis; (type of intake, amount of pure ethanol taken per day in grams, n=number of human subjects). Y-axis; PEth concentration (µmol/liter whole blood, mean ± SD).

detectable PEth for 7 days or more after having ended drinking (table 1), and it was concluded that PEth had a half-life of about 4 days (Varga et al., 2000). Since PEth normally is zero, one could expect PEth being normalized after 1 - 2 weeks in individuals having PEth less than 10 µmol/l, and after 2 - 3 weeks in individuals having PEth above 10 µmol/l (Varga et al., 2000).

Pat nr	Day 1 PEth (µmol/L)	Day 3 PEth (µmol/L)	Day 5 PEth (µmol/L)	Day 7 PEth (µmol/L)
1	0	0	-	0
2	9.4	7.0	5.0	4.1
3	0	0	-	0
4	1.2	0.8	-	-
5	2.7	1.8	-	0
6	17.8	9.3	-	7.5
7	8.0	5.6	3.2	3.1
8	7.7	4.7	3.6	1.8
9	3.2	2.1	1.3	-
10	4.8	2.7	3.2	-
11	10.9	7.4	6.0	4.1
12	4.3	3.3	1.8	1.6
13	3.9	3.2	2.3	0.9
14	0	0	0	0
15	2.7	1.4	1.1	0.9

Table 1 Decline of Phosphatidylethanol (PEth; in µmol/liter whole blood) concentrations in blood of 15 chronic alcoholics during detoxification as inpatients. Time of sampling (day 1 = first day of sobriety).

4. Conclusions

PEth is an abnormal phospholipid, formed in mammalian cells only in the presence of ethanol. The formation of PEth is catalysed by PLD. During the last few years, research and publications on PLDs has exploded. Excellent reviews have recently been published, each with hundreds of references (Cockroft 1997, Exton 1999, Frohman et al. 1999, Meier et al. 1999, Liscovitch et al. 1999, Liscovitch et al 2000). Not much of this new knowledge concern the formation of PEth, but it is now evident that primary alcohols, like ethanol, are excellent substrates for PLD and preferred over water, the actual substrate in vivo, by at least 1000-fold. The degradation rate for PEth seems to vary among organs and cells and to be especially slow in erythrocytes.

Encouraged by our findings of PEth in neutrophils from a few alcoholics, we designed studies to search for PEth in whole blood from alcohol exposed persons.

The assay system has developed from thin-layer chromatography and time consuming quantitative determinations to HPLC-ELSD that operates with an autosampler. Identification of PEth molecules has applied mass spectrometry. Analytical interference of drugs used by alcoholics has been checked for. Studies on cellular distribution in blood has revealed that almost all PEth is confined to erythrocytes and almost nothing in white blood cells or plasma.

Based on findings in alcohol drinking volunteers we conclude that a single dose of ethanol (32 - 47 g) does not produce measurable amounts of PEth, but a three week load of 750 - 1000 g (40 - 50 g daily) seemed to be required to create PEth that could be measured. In alcoholics the highest level of PEth was 10 times higher than ever found in volunteers. PEth is a new and promising marker for alcohol abuse in view of its high biological specificity.

References

Albani-Torregrossa S., Attucci S., Marinozzi M., Pelliciarri R., Moroni F. and Pellegrini-Giampietro D.E. (1999) Antagonist pharmacology of metabotropic glutamate receptors coupled to phospholipase D activation in adult rat hippocampus; focus on (2R,1′S,2′R,3′S)-2-(2′-carboxy-3′-phenylcyclopropyl)glycine versus 3,5-dihydroxyphenylglycine. Molecular Pharmacology 55, 699-707.

Alling C., Gustavsson L. and Änggård E. (1983) An abnormal phospholipid in rat organs after ethanol. FEBS Letters 152 24-28.

Alling C., Gustavsson L., Månsson J., Benthi G. and Änggård E. (1984) Phosphatidylethanol formation in rat organs after ethanol treatment. Biochimica et Biophysica Acta 793, 119-122.

Alling C., Gustavsson L., Larsson C., Lundqvist C., Rodriguez D. and Simonsson P (1994) Adaptation of signal transduction in brain. In: Towards a Molecular Basis of Alcóhol Use and Abuse (eds) Jansson B., Jörnvall H., Rydberg U., Terenius L. and Vallee, B. L. Birkhäuser Verlag, Basel, Switzerland, pp. 19-28.

Asaoka Y., Kikkawa U., Sekiguchi K., Shearman M. S., Kosaka Y., Nakano Y., Satoh T. and Nishizuka Y. (1988) Activation of a brain-specific protein kinase C subspecies in the presence of phosphatidylethanol. FEBS Letters 231, 221-224.

Billah M.M. (1993) Phospholipase D and cell signaling. Current Opinion in Immunology 5, 114-123.

Billah M. M. and Anthes J. C. (1990) The regulation and cellular functions of phosphatidylcholine hydrolysis. Biochemical Journal 269, 281-291.

Boarder M.R. (1994) A role for phospholipase D in control of mitogenesis. Trends in Pharmacological Sciences 15, 57-62.

Bondeson J. and Sundler R. (1987) Phosphatidylethanol counteracts calcium-induced membrane fusion but promotes proton-induced fusion. Biochimica et Biophysica Acta 899, 258-264.

Boyano-Adánez M.C. and Gustavsson L. (1993) Effects of ethanol on receptor-mediated phospholipase D activity in human neuroblastoma cells. In: Alcohol, Cell membranes and Signal Transduction in Brain 265-272. (Eds. Alling C., Diamond I., Leslie S., Sun G.Y. and Wood W.G., New York, Plenum Press).

Boyano-Adánez M.C., Rodríguez F. D., Aradóttir S., Alling C. and Gustavsson L. (1994) Protein kinase C-mediated phospholipase D activity is increased by linolenic acid supplementation in NG108-15 cells. Biochemica et Biophysica Acta 1214, 263-271.

Boyano-Adánez M.C., Lundqvist C., Larsson C. and Gustavsson L. (1997) Characterization of phospholipase D activation by muscarinic receptors in human neuroblastoma SH-SY 5Y cells. Neuropharmacology 36, 295-304.

Brindley D.N., Waggoner D.W. (1998) Mammalian lipid phosphate phosphohydrolases. Journal of Biological Chemistry 273, 24281-24284.

Brown F..D., Thompson N., Saqib K.M., Clark J.M., Powner D., Thompson N.T., Solari R. and Wakelam M.J.O. (1998) Phospholipase D1 localises to secretory granules and lysosomes and is plasma-membrane translocated on cellular stimulation. Current Biology 8, 835-838.

Brown H.A. and Sternweis, P.C. (1995) Stimulation of phospholipase D by ADP-ribosylation factors. Methods of Enzymology 257, 313-324.

Browning J. L. (1981) Motions and interactions of phospholipid head groups at the membrane surface. 1. Simple alkyl head groups. Biochemistry 20, 7123-7133.

Cockcroft S. (1997) Phospholipase D: Regulation by GTPases and protein kinase C and physiological relevance. Progress in Lipid Research 35, 345-370.

Colley W.C., Altschuller Y.M., Sue-Ling C.K., Copeland, N.G., Gilbert D.J., Jenkins N.A., Branch K.D., Tsirka S.E., Bollag R.G., Bollag W.B. and Frohman M.A. (1997a) Cloning and expression analysis of murine phospholipase D1. Biochemical Journal. 326, 745-753.

Colley W.C., Sung T.C, Roll R., Jenco J., Hammond S.M., Altschuller Y., Bar-Sagi D., Morris A.J. and Frohman M.A. (1997b). Phospholipase D2, a distinct phospholipase D isoform with novel regulatory properties that provokes cytoskeletal reorganization. Current Biology 7, 191-201.

Cross M.J., Roberts. S., Ridley A.J., Hodgkin M.N., Stewart A., Claesson-Welsh L, Wakelam M.J.O. (1996) Stimulation of actin stress fibre formation mediated by activation of phospholipase D. Current Biology 5, 588-597.

Czarny M., Fiucci G., Lavie Y., Banno Y., Nozawa Y. and Liscovitch M. (2000). Phospholipase D2: functional interaction with caveolin in low-density membrane microdomains. FEBS Letters 467, 326-332.

Daniel L.W., Huan C., Strum J.C., Smitherman P. K., Greene. D. and Wykle R. L. (1993) Phospholipase D hydrolysis of choline phosphoglycerides is selective for the alkyl-linked subclass of Madin-Darby canine kidney cells. Journal of Biological Chemistry 268, 21519-21526.

Dawson R. M. C. (1967) The formation of phosphatidylglycerol and other phospholipids by the transferase activity of phospholipase D. Biochemical Journal 102, 205-210.

Exton J.H. (1994) Phosphatidylcholine breakdown and signal transduction. Biochimica et Biophysica Acta 1212, 26-42.

Exton J.H. (1997) New developments in phospholipase D. Journal of Biological Chemistry 272, 15579-15582.

Exton J.H. (1998) Phospholipase D. Biochemica et Biophysica Acta 1436, 105-115.

Exton J. H. (1999) Regulation of phospholipase D. Biochimica et Biophysica Acta 1439, 121-133.

Frohman M. A., Sung T.-C. and Morris A. J. (1999) Mammalian phospholipase D structure and regulation. Biochimica et Biophysica Acta 1439, 175-186.

Gatalica Z., Moehren G. and Hoek J. B. (1993) Unilateral nephrectomy selectively stimulates phospholipase D in the remaining kidney. Biochimica et Biophysica Acta. 1177, 87-92.

Gruchalla R. S., Dinh T. T. and Kennerly D. A. (1990) An indirect pathway of receptor-mediated 1,2-diacylglycerol formation in mast cells. I. IgE receptor-mediated activation of phospholipase D. Journal of Immunology 144, 2334-2342.

Gunnarsson T., Karlsson A., Hansson P., Johnson G., Alling C. and Odham G. (1998) Determination of phosphatidylethanol in blood from alcoholic males using high-performance liquid chromatography and evaporative light scattering of electrospray mass spectrometric detection. Journal of Chromatography B 705, 243-249.

Gustavsson L. (1995) Phosphatidylethanol formation: Specific effects of ethanol mediated via phospholipase D. Alcohol and Alcoholism 30, 391-406.

Gustavsson L. and Alling C. (1987) Formation of phosphatidylethanol in rat brain by phospholipase D. Biochemical and Biophysical Research Communications 142, 958-963.

Gustavsson L. and Hansson E. (1990) Stimulation of phospholipase D activity by phorbol esters in cultured astrocytes. Journal of Neurochemistry 54, 737-742.

Hammond S.M., Altschuller Y.M., Sung T.C., Rudge S.A., Rose K, Engebrecht J, Morris A.J. and Frohman M.A. (1995). Human ADP-ribosylating factor-activated phosphatidylcholine-specific phospholipase D defines a new and highly conserved gene family. Journal of Biological Chemistry 270, 29640-29643.

Hammond S. M., Jenco J. M., Nakashima S., Cadwallader K., Gu Q.-M., Cook S., Nozawa Y., Prestwick G. D., Frohman M. A. and Morris A. J. (1997) Characterization of two alternatively spliced forms of phospholipase D1. Activation of the purified enzymes by phosphatidylinositol 4,5-bisphosphate, ADP-ribosylation factor, and Rho family monomeric GTP-binding proteins and protein kinase C-α. Journal of Biological Chemistry 272, 3860-3868.

Han J.S., Kim H.C., Chung J.K, Kang H.S., Donaldson J.and Koh, J.K (1998) The potential role for CDC42 protein from rat brain cytosol in phospholipase D activation. Biochem. Mol. Biol. Int 45, 1089-1103.

Hansson P., Caron M., Johnson G., Gustavsson L and Alling C. (1997) Blood phosphatidylethanol as a marker of alcoholic abuse: Levels in alcoholic males during withdrawal Alcoholism: Clinical and Experimental Research 21, 108-110.

Heller M. (1978) Phospholipase D. Advances in Lipid Research 16, 267-326.

Hii C. S.T., Kokke Y. S., Pruimboom W. and Murray A. W. (1989) Phorbol esters stimulate a phospholipase D-catalysed reaction with both ester- and ether-linked phospholipids in HeLa cells. FEBS Letters 257, 35-37.

Holbrook P. G., Pannell L. K., Murata Y. and Daly J. W. (1992) Molecular species analysis of a product of phospholipase D activation. Journal of Biological Chemistry 267, 16834-16840.

Horwitz J. (1991) Bradykinin activates a phospholipase D that hydrolyzes phosphatidylcholine in PC12 cells. Journal of Neurochemistry 56, 509-517.

Kanaho Y., Kanoh H., Saitoh K. and Nozawa Y. (1991) Phospholipase D activation by platelet-activating factor, leukotriene B4, and formyl-methionyl-leucyl-phenylalanine in rabbit neutrophils. Phospholipase D activation is involved in enzyme release. Journal of Immunology 146, 3536-3541.

Kanfer J.N. (1980) The base-exchange enzymes and phospholipase D of mammalian tissue. Can. J. Biochem. 58, 1370-1380.

Katayama K., Kodaki T., Nagamachi Y. andYamashita S. (1998) Cloning, differential regulation and tissue distribution of ADP-ribosylating factor-dependent phospholipase D from rat liver. Biochemical Journal 299, 109-114.

Kiss Z. (1996) Regulation of phospholipase D by protein kinase C. Chem. Phys. Lipids 80, 81-102.
Kobayashi M. and Kanfer J. (1987) Phosphatidylethanol formation via transphosphatidylation by rat brain synaptosomal phospholipase D. Journal of Neurochemistry 48, 1597-1603.
Kodaki T. and Yamashita S. (1997) Cloning, expression and characterization of a novel phospholipase D complementary DNA from rat brain. Journal of Biological Chemistry 272, 11408-11413.
Konishi F., Kondo T. and Inagami T. (1991) Phospholipase D in cultured rat vascular smooth muscle cells and its activation by phorbol ester. Biochemical and Biophysical Research Communications 179, 1070-1076.
Kötter K. and Klein J. (1999) Ethanol inhibits astroglial cell proliferation by disruption of phospholipase D-mediated signaling. Journal of Neurochemistry 73, 2517-2523.
Ktistakis N. T., Brown H. A., Water M., Sternweis P. C. and Roth M. G. (1996) Evidence that phospholipase D mediates ADP ribosylation factor-dependent formation of Golgi coated vesicles. Journal of Cell Biology 134, 295-306.
Lee M. and Bell R. M. (1992) Supplementation of the phosphatidyl-L-serine requirements of protein kinase C with nonactivating phospholipids. Biochemistry 31, 5176-5182.
Lieber C. S. (1995) Medical disorders of alcoholism. New England Journal of Medicine 333, 1058-1065.
Lin P. Y., Wiggan G. A. and Gilfillan A. M. (1991) Activation of phospholipase-D in a rat mast (RBL-2H3) cell line – a possible unifying mechanism for IgE-dependent degranulation and arachidonic acid metabolite release. Journal of Immunology 146, 1609-1616.
Liscovitch M., Chalifa V., Pertile P., Chen C. S. and Cantley L. C. (1994) Novel function of phosphatidyl inositol 4,5 bisphosphate as a cofactor for brain membrane phospholipase D. Journal of Biological Chemistry 269, 21403-21406.
Liscovitch M., Czarny M., Fiucci G., Lavie Y., Tang X. (1999) Localization and possible functions of phospholipase D isozymes. Biochimica et Biophysica Acta 1439, 245-263.
Liscovitch M., Czarny M., Fiucci G. and Tang X. (2000) Phospholipase D: molecular and cell biology of a novel gene family. Biochemical Journal 345, 401-415.
Lopez I., Burns D. J., Lambeth J. D. (1995) Regulation of phospholipase D by protein kinase C in human neutrophils. Conventional isoforms of protein kinasc C phosphorylate a phospholipase D-related component in the plasma membrane. Journal of Biological Chemistry 270, 19465-19472.
Lopez I., Arnold R. S. and Lambeth J. D. (1998) Cloning and initial characterization of a human phospholipase D2 (hPLD2), ADP-ribosylation factor regulates hPLD2. Journal of Biological Chemistry 273, 12846-12852.
Lundqvist C., Rodríguez F. D., Simonsson P., Alling C. and Gustavsson L. (1993) Phosphatidylethanol affects inositol 1,4,5-trisphosphate levels in NG108-15 neuroblastoma x glioma hybrid cells. Journal of Neurochemistry 60, 738-744.
Lundqvist C., Alling C., Aradóttir S. and Gustavsson L. (1994a) Agonist-stimulated phospholipase D-activity and phosphatidylethanol accumulation in neutrophils from alcoholics. Alcoholism: Clinical and Experimental Research 18, 580-586.
Lundqvist C, Aradóttir S., Alling C., Boyano-Adenez M. C. and Gustavsson L. (1994b) Phosphatidylethanol formation and degradation in brains of acutely and repeatedly ethanol-treated rats. Neuroscience Letters 179, 127-131.
Luo J Q., Liu X., Frankel, Rotunda T., Ramos M., Flom J., Jiang H., Feig L. A., Morris A. J., Kahn R. A. and Foster D. A. (1998) Functional association between Arf and RalA in active phospholipase D complex. Proceedings of the National Academy of Sciences USA 95, 3632-3637.
Malcolm K.C., Ross A.H., Qiu R.G., Symons M. and Exton J.H. (1994) Activation of rat liver phospholipase D by the small GTP-binding protein RhoA. Journal of Biological Chemistry 269, 25951-25954.
Meier K. E., Gibbs T. C., Knoepp S. M. and Ella K. M. (1999) Expression of phospholipase D isoforms in mammalian cells. Biochimica et Biophysica Acta 1439, 199-213.
Metz S. A. and Dunlop M. (1990) Production of phosphatidylethanol by phospholipase D phosphatidyl transferase in intact or dispersed pancreatic islets: evidence for the in situ metabolism of phosphatidylethanol. Archives of Biochemistry and Biophysics 283, 417-428.
Mitchell R., McCulloch D., Lutz E., Johnson M., NacKenzie C., Fennell M., Fink G., Zhou W. and Sealfon S.C. (1998) Rhodopsin-family receptors associate with small G proteins to activate phospholipase D. Nature 392, 411-414.
Min D.S., Park S.K, Exton J.H. (1998) Characterization of a rat brain phospholipase D isozyme. Journal of Biological Chemistry 273, 7044-7051.
Mizunuma M., Tanaka S., Kudo R. and Kanoh H. (1993) Phospholipase D activity of human amnion cells stimulated with phorbol ester and bradykinin. Biochimica et Biophysica Acta 1168, 213-219.

Moehren G., Gustavsson L. and Hoek J. B. (1994) Activation and desensitization of phospholipase D in intact rat hepatocytes. Journal of Biological Chemistry 283, 838-848.

Moolenaar W.H. (1995) Lysophosphatidic acid, a multifunctional phospholipid messenger. Journal of Biological Chemistry 270, 12949-12952.

Morris A.J., Engebrecht J., Ohguchi K., Banno Y., Nakashima S. and Nozawa Y (1996) Regulation of membrane-bound phosholipase D by protein kinase C in HL-60 cells. Synergistic action of small GTP-binding protein RhoA. Journal of Biological Chemistry 271, 4366-4372.

Omodeo-Salé M. F., Cestaro B., Mascherpa A., Monti D. and Masserini M. (1989) Enzymatic synthesis and thermotropic behaviour of phosphatidylethanol. Chemistry and Physics of Lipids 50, 135-142.

Omodeo-Salé M. F., Lindi C., Palestini P. and Masserini M. (1991) Role of phosphatidylethanol in membranes – effects on membrane fluidity, tolerance to ethanol, and activity of membrane-bound enzymes. Biochemistry 30, 2477-2482.

Pai J., Liebl E. C., Tettenborn C. S., Ikegwuonu F. I. and Mueller G. C. (1987) 12-O-Tetradecanoyl-phorbol-13-acetate activates the synthesis of phosphatidylethanol in animal cells exposed to ethanol. Carcinogenesis 8, 173-178.

Park S.K., Provost J..J,, Dae Bae C., Ho W.T. and Exton J.H. (1997) Cloning and characterization of phospholipase D from rat brain. Journal of Biological Chemistry 272, 29263-29271.

Pedersen K.M., Finsen B. Celis J.E. and Jensen N.A. (1998) Expression of a novel murine phospholipase D homolog coincides with late neuronal development in the forebrain. Journal of Biological Chemistry 273, 31494-31504.

Purkiss J. R. (1994) Effect of incorporation of phosphatidylethanol on release of noradrenaline from SHSY5Y human neuroblastoma cells. British Journal of Pharmacology 112, 321P.

Rodríguez F. D., Lundqvist C., Gustavsson L. and Alling C. (1994) Chronic ethanol treatment reduces the binding of [3H]-inositol 1,4,5 trisphosphate to rat cerebellar membranes. Pharmacology and Toxicology 74, 34.

Rodríguez F. D., Lundqvist C., Alling C. and Gustavsson L. (1996) Ethanol and phosphatidylethanol reduce the binding of [3H]-inositol 1,4,5 trisphosphate to rat cerebellar membranes. Alcohol and Alcoholism 31, 453-461.

Roth M.G., Bi K., Ktistakis N.T. and Yu S. (1999) Phospholipase D as an effector for ADP-ribosylation factor in the regulation of vesicular traffic. Chemistry and Physics of Lipids 98, 141-152.

Rottenberg H., Bittman R. and Li H. (1992) Resistance to ethanol disordering of membranes from ethanol-fed rats is conferred by all phospholipid classes. Biochimica et Biophysica Acta 1123, 282-290.

SarriE., Servitj J.-M., Picatoste F. and Claro E. (1996) Two phosphatidylethanol classes separated by thin layer chromatography are produced by phospholipase D in rat brain hippocampal slices. FEBS Letters 393, 303-306.

Sciorra V.A., Rudge S.A., Prestwich G.D. Frohman M.A., Engebrecht J. And Morris A.J. (1999) Identification of a phosphoinositide binding motif that mediates activation of mammalian and yeast phospholipase D isoenzymes. EMBO Journal 18, 5911-5921.

Seidler L., Kaszkin M. and Kinzel V. (1996) Primary alcohols and phosphatidylcholine metabolism in rat brain synaptosomal membranes via phospholipase D. Pharmacology and Toxicology 78, 249-253.

Shukla S. D. and Halenda S. P. (1991) Phospholipase D in cells signalling and its relationship to phospholipase C. Life Sciences 48, 851-866.

Singer W. D., Brown H. A., Bokoch G. M. and Sternweis P. C. (1995) Resolved phospholipase D activity is modulated by cytosolic factors other than Arf. Journal of Biological Chemistry 270, 14944-14950.

Slaaby R., Jensen T., Hansen H.S., Frohman M.A. and Seedorf K. (1998) PLD2 complexes with the EGF receptor and undergoes tyrosine phosphorylation at a single site upon agonist stimulation. Journal of Biological Chemistry 273, 33722-33727.

Steed P.M. Clark K.L., Boyar W.C., Lasala D.J. (1998) Charcterization of human PLD2 and the analysis of PLD isoform splice variants. FASEB Journal 12, 1309-1317.

Suju M., Davila M., Poleo G., Docampo R. and Benaim G. (1996) Phosphatidylethanol stimulates the plasma-membrane calcium pump from human erythrocytes. Biochemical Journal 317, 933-938.

Sun G. Y., Huang H.-M., Lee D. Z. and Sun A. Y. (1984) Increased acid phospholipids in rat brain membranes after chronic ethanol administration. Life Sciences 35, 2127-2133.

Sung T.C., Zhang Y., Morris A.J. and Frohman M.A.(1999) Structural analysis of human PLD2. Journal of Biological Chemistry 274, 3659-3666.

Thompson N. T., Garland L. G. and Bonser R. W. (1993) Phospholipase D: regulation and functional significance. Advances in Pharmacology 24, 199-238.

Tomic S., Greiser U., Lammers R., Kharitonenkov A., Imyanitov E., Ullrich A. and Bohmer F.D. (1995) Association of SH2 domain protein tyrosine phsophatases with the epidermal growth factor receptor in human tumor cells. Phosphatidic acid activates receptor dephosphorylation by PTP1C. Journal of Biological Chemistry 270, 21277-21284.

Topham M.K. and Prescott S.M. (1998) Structural analysis of human PLD1. Journal of Biological Chemistry 274, 11447-11450.

Tou J.-S., Xu M. and Wang F. (1999) Formation of phosphatidic acid and subclasses of phosphatidylethanol in human neutrophils upon interleukin-8 stimulation. Cellular Signalling 11, 137-141.

Wang P., Anthes J. C., Siegel I. M., Egan R. W. and Billah M. M. (1991) Existence of cytosolic phospholipase D. Identification and comparison with membrane-bound enzyme. Journal of Biological Chemistry 266, 14877-14880.

Varga A., Hansson P., Lundqvist C. and Alling C. (1998) Phosphatidylethanol in blood as a marker of ethanol consumption in healthy volunteers: Comparison with other markers. Alcoholism: Clinical and Experimental Research 22, 1832-1837.

Varga A., Hansson P., Johnson G. and Alling C. (2000) Normalization rate and cellular localization of phosphatidylethanol in whole blood from chronic alcoholics. Clinica Chimica Acta 299, 141-150.

Victorov A. V., Janes N., Moehren G., Rubin E., Taraschi T. and Hoek J. B. (1994) Rapid transbilayer movement of phosphatidylethanol in unilamellar phosphatidylcholine vesicles. Journal of the American Chemical Society 116, 4050-4052.

Vinggard A. M. and Hansen H. S. (1993) Bradykinin and vasopressin activate phospholipase D in rat Leydig cells by a protein kinase C-dependent mechanism. Journal of Endocrinology 136, 119-126.

Yang S. F., Freer S. and Benson A. A. (1967) Transphosphatidylation by phospholipase D. Journal of Biological Chemistry 242, 477-484.

Yu C.-H., Liu S.-Y. and Panagia V. (1996) The transphosphatidylation activity of phospholipase D. Molecular and Cellular Biochemistry 157, 101-105.

Zhang Y., Altschuller Y.M., Hammond S.M., Hayes F., Morris A.J. and Frohman M.A. (1999) Loss of recptor regulation by phospholipase D1 mutant unresponsive to protein kinase C. EMBO Journal 18, 6339-6348.

Zhang W., Nakashima T., Saka N., Yamada H., Okano Y. and Nozawa Y. (1992) Activation of phospholipase D by platelet-derived growth factor (PDGF) in rat C6 glioma cells. Possible role in mitogenic signal transduction. Neurological Research 14, 397-401.

Proteins modified by direct and indirect ethanol metabolites, and their associated antibodies, as markers of alcohol intake

Simon Worrall

Alcohol Research Unit
Department of Biochemistry
University of Queensland
QLD 4072
Australia

Phone: +61-7-3365 4626
FAX: +61-7-3365 4699
Email: worrall@biosci.uq.edu.au

Introduction

Alcohol is the most widely abused drug in Western societies. As such it is a significant cause of morbidity and mortality, costing Australia about AU$ 8 billion in 1992 (Collins and Lapsley, 1996). However, there are two sides to drinking which need to be disentangled. It is generally accepted that low alcohol intake (20 - 40g ethanol/day for males; 20g/day for females) is beneficial, protecting against coronary heart disease, a major killer of the middle-aged. However, high intake (> 100g ethanol/day) has a series of adverse effects which include liver disease, brain damage, heart and skeletal muscle wasting (Collins and Lapsley, 1996). Thus, it is important to have a reliable clinical measure of alcohol intake to detect those people that have hazardous levels of drinking.

Over the past 20 - 30 years many markers have been used as a measure of alcohol intake. The majority of these markers, for example serum transaminase activities, are not totally specific for alcohol abuse and only become elevated when alcohol intake is very high. Ideally a test that is specific for alcohol and would detect people with lower but still hazardous alcohol intake is required. This has lead to an intensive search for better markers over the last 10 - 20 years. The best "new" marker to be developed is carbohydrate-deficient transferrin (CDT; Stibler and Hultcrantz, 1987) though it has recently been criticised for a lack of specificity for alcohol abuse and is not particularly useful for detecting hazardous drinking (see, for example Sarkola et al., 2000).

The oxidation of ethanol, mainly by the liver, produces a series of metabolites that can readily react with macromolecules to produce both stable and unstable covalent adducts. It was originally proposed that these modified proteins could be used as a marker of alcohol intake in a manner analogous to the use of glycated haemoglobin as an indicator of glucose levels in diabetics. However, this has proven to be more difficult than was previously imagined. Many researchers have shown that these modified proteins are immunogenic, leading to the generation of antibodies which react with the modifications per se and with the carrier protein (Niemela et al., 1987; Hoerner et al., 1988; Worrall et al., 1989). Thus, it has been proposed by myself and others that measurement of antibody reactivity with modified proteins may also be useful to detect chronic alcohol abuse.

This chapter will cover the work which has been carried out on the detection and measurement of modified proteins and their associated antibodies in drinkers, will look at the utility of modified proteins or anti-modification antibodies as markers of hazardous and high alcohol intake, and will discuss the problems that are limiting developments in this area. Furthermore, this chapter is not intended as an exhaustive review of the literature but will highlight significant advances in this area of research.

Alcohol metabolism and the generation of reactive metabolites

Imbibed ethanol is readily absorbed from the stomach and intestine. Some of the ethanol is metabolised by the stomach (~10 %) but the majority is delivered to the liver via the hepatic portal vein and then enters the systemic circulation. The liver is the major site of ethanol metabolism (Lieber, 2000), being able to oxidise about 10 - 15g/hr. Hepatic oxidation is largely confined to hepatocytes (the main cell type) and is carried out by two main systems (Figure 1). The first is alcohol dehydrogenase that is located in the cytosol and is of major importance when blood alcohol levels are low. The second is the microsomal ethanol oxidising system (MEOS) which is sited in the smooth endoplasmic reticulum and has a low affinity for ethanol (see review by Lieber, 1999). This is the major oxidising system when blood alcohol levels are high. On prolonged drinking this system is inducible and in a consistently heavy drinking person accounts for up to 70 % of ethanol metabolism. Both alcohol dehydrogenase and MEOS oxidise ethanol to acetaldehyde. Acetaldehyde is a highly reactive species which would lead to cellular damage if a significant amount accumulated. To prevent this the acetaldehyde is oxidised to acetic acid by a family of aldehyde dehydrogenase enzymes that are present in the mitochondria and the cytoplasm.

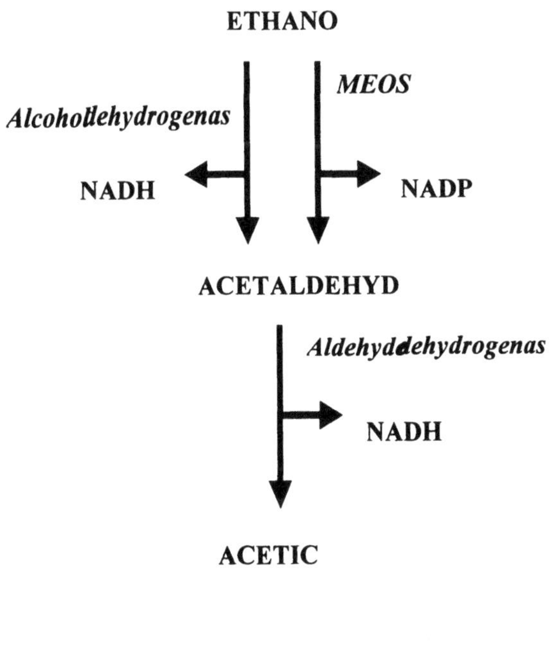

Figure 1 The main pathways of ethanol oxidation

MEOS, as well as producing acetaldehyde, also produces as series of free radicals such as α-hydroxyethyl and hydroxyl radicals which can lead to cellular damage by reaction with proteins and unsaturated fatty acids in biological membranes. The attack on membranes by free radicals leads to lipid peroxidation and generates the reactive aldehydes, malondialdehyde and 4-hydroxynonenal, by the cleavage of lipid peroxides. In this chapter I shall refer to acetaldehyde and α-hydroxyethyl radicals as direct metabolites, and malondialdehyde and 4-hydroxynonenal as indirect metabolites.

Evidence for protein modification as a result of ethanol metabolism

Many in vitro studies have shown that metabolites produced during ethanol oxidation react with macromolecules such as proteins to produce both stable and unstable covalent adducts. These studies have been useful in identifying some proteins as potential targets for metabolically-derived reactive species. A lot of basic information about the chemistry of metabolite-protein interactions has been obtained from such studies. The chemistry of adduct formation is beyond the scope of this review but several good reviews are available for acetaldehyde (Nicholls et al., 1992; Tuma and Sorrell, 1995) and malondialdehyde (Esterbauer et al., 1991) and 4-hydroxynonenal (Esterbauer et al., 1991) adducts.

A considerable body of evidence exists to demonstrate that metabolite-modified proteins are generated during the metabolism of ethanol within the liver. Initial studies, using cell-free liver homogenates (Donohue et al., 1983) and liver slices (Medina et al., 1985), showed that acetaldehyde generated during ethanol oxidation reacted with hepatic proteins to produce acetaldehyde-protein adducts. It also appeared that unstable adducts were initially formed, and were then stabilized during more prolonged incubation to produce stable products. More direct evidence of adduct formation came after polyclonal antisera raised against proteins modified by acetaldehyde in vitro were used in Western and immunohistochemical analysis of liver samples from rodents fed ethanol and human alcoholics. However, while all of these studies found that acetaldehyde had reacted with hepatic protein(s), the number and cellular location of the protein targets was very different in each study. Two studies detected single modified proteins. Behrens et al. (1988) found that cytochrome P4502E1 (an enzyme which is part of MEOS and oxidizes ethanol to acetaldehyde) in the endoplasmic reticulum was modified whereas Lin et al. (1988) could only detect a 37 kDa cytosolic protein (later identified as Δ^4-3-ketosteroid-5β reductase (Zhu et al., 1996)). In contrast Worrall et al. (1991 b) and Yokoyama et al. (1993) detected multiple modified cytosolic proteins, including the 37 kDa one seen by Lin et al. Furthermore, Nicholls et al. (1994), using ELISAs, demonstrated the presence of modified proteins in hepatic cytosol, membrane and mitochondrial fractions from ethanol-fed rats. They went on to show that cytosolic α-tubulin, glyceraldehyde-3-phosphate dehydrogenase, calmodulin and a series of other proteins carried acetaldehyde-derived modifications (Nicholls, de Jersey, Wilce and Worrall, unpublished results). Niemela and coworkers (1991 b) used immunohistochemistry to demonstrate modified proteins in the cytosol of hepatocytes from human alcoholics. Further studies have shown that acetaldehyde-modified epitopes are located in the cytoplasm and are more intense in the centrilobular regions of the liver (Holstege et al., 1994; Paradis et al., 1996), the areas associated with the highest levels of ethanol oxidation. The studies using rodents have been useful in the study of adduct formation as it has been shown that antibodies from human alcoholics react with cytosolic proteins from ethanol-fed but not control rats, suggesting that similar, if not identical, immunogenic epitopes are being generated (Worrall et al., 1994).

Much less work has been done on the other metabolites. α-Hydroxyethyl radicals have been shown to be produced during ethanol oxidation by CYP2E1 (Albano et al., 1988) and to react with microsomal and other proteins. Hydroxyethyl radical-modified proteins have been detected in tissues from ethanol-fed rats (Iimuro et al., 1996) and human alcoholics (Clot et al., 1996). Malondialdehyde and 4-hydroxynonenal are the major products of the oxidative degradation (peroxidation) of polyunsaturated fatty acids. Elevated levels of malondialdehyde have been detected in humans drinking about 100g of ethanol per day (Clot et al., 1994). The increase in malondialdehyde production appears to continue for several weeks after cessation of drinking (Lecomte et al., 1994). Malondialdehyde and 4-hydroxynonenal have been shown by numerous groups to react with proteins in vitro to produce a variety of different adducts. Malondialdehyde-modified proteins have been detected in vivo in a wide range of conditions. For example, hepatic cytosol and plasma from rats with hepatic iron overload contained elevated levels of malondialdehyde-and 4-hydroxynonenal-protein adducts (Houglum et al., 1990). In animal models of alcoholic liver disease several researchers have shown that 4-hydroxynonenal- and malondialdehyde-modified proteins are associated with areas of inflammation and necrosis (Kamimura et al., 1992; Niemela et al., 1995; Li et al., 1997; Niemela et al., 1998). Furthermore, Ohhira and coworkers (Ohhira et al., 1998) have recently shown that 4-hydroxynonenal-modified proteins are associated with iron deposits in hepatocytes, and appear to be a marker of oxidative stress-induced damage.

More recently a new family of adducts have been identified which are derived from acetaldehyde and malondialdehyde reacting in concert to produce modifications which contain both acetaldehyde and malondialdehyde. These hybrid adducts were termed MAlondialdehyde-Acetaldehyde (MAA) adducts by Tuma and coworkers (Tuma et al., 1996). Two major forms of MAA adducts have now been identified as 4-methyl-1,4-dihydropyridine-3,5-dicarbaldehyde (MAA 2:1, derived from two molecules of malondialdehyde and one molecule of acetaldehyde) and 2-formyl-3-(alkylamino)butanal (MAA 1:1, derived from one molecule of acetaldehyde and one molecule of malondialdehyde) derivatives of protein amino groups (Tuma et al., 1996; Kearley et al., 1999). Polyclonal antibodies have been generated against MAA 2:1 and have been used to show that these adducts are formed in the liver of ethanol-fed rats (Tuma et al., 1996; Xu et al., 1997; Worrall et al., 2000). There is now evidence to suggest that MAA 1:1 adducts react with malondialdehyde-derived Schiff bases to form the MAA 2:1 adduct (Tuma et al., 2001). The MAA 2:1 adduct is unique in that it makes carrier proteins immuno genic in the absence of adjuvant (Thiele et al., 1998) and may therefore play an important role in the aetiology of tissue damage associated with alcohol abuse.

Can proteins modified by ethanol metabolites be used as a marker of alcohol intake?

After alcohol ingestion some acetaldehyde generated during ethanol oxidation is released from the liver into the circulation. This acetaldehyde can reversibly bind to red cells and plasma proteins and travel to extrahepatic tissues (Baraona et al., 1987a; b). Many researchers have measured modified plasma proteins and haemoglobin to see whether either of these measurements could act as a marker of alcohol intake.

The concentration of circulating proteins modified by acetaldehyde has been measured in two studies, both of which used ELISA technology. Lin and coworkers (Lin et al., 1990) were able to demonstrate larger amounts of acetaldehyde-modified serum proteins in samples from alcoholics than teetotal controls. Interestingly in this study a clearer differentiation between alcoholic and controls was seen if an antiserum raised against acetaldehyde-modified myoglobin rather than modified haemocyanin was used. The reasons for this discrepancy are not clear but it is possible that the myoglobin acts as a carrier protein to make adducts more representative of serum proteins than does haemocyanin. In a more recent study (Worrall et al., 1998) we were able to show that alcoholics had statistically significantly higher levels of acetaldehyde-modified albumin than heavy drinkers or control social drinkers. Furthermore, the heavy drinkers had higher levels than the controls. These data suggest that the level of acetaldehyde-modified albumin is related to the amount of alcohol consumed. Albumin was chosen in our study because we believed that it would be more representative of liver acetaldehyde concentrations since it is synthesized within the liver and then secreted into the circulation. Thus, it has the opportunity to be modified during its synthesis and secretion, as well as when in the bloodstream. In rats fed ethanol we have shown that albumin and IgG (a protein of extrahepatic origin) are both modified by acetaldehyde suggesting that modification also takes place outside of the liver (Worrall et al., 2000).

Most of the effort on the measurement of modified proteins has centred on the modification of haemoglobin by acetaldehyde. Early studies on the reactivity of acetaldehyde with purified proteins in vitro had shown that acetaldehyde readily reacts with numerous sites on the globin monomers, particularly at the amino terminus of the β-chain (San George and Hoberman, 1986). The initial studies on the isolation and characterization of acetaldehyde-modified haemoglobin from alcoholic blood were unsuccessful (see for example (Stockham and Blanke, 1988)). However, Niemela et al. (1990) used an ELISA to detect acetaldehyde-modified haemoglobin in the blood of volunteers after acute dosing at 1.3 - 2.9 g of ethanol per Kg body weight over 8 hr. Using a similar ELISA, they (Niemela et al., 1991a) were also able to show that acetaldehyde-modified haemoglobin levels were higher in women who subsequently delivered children with foetal alcohol effects than those who delivered normal children. In addition, the same technique also showed that the level of modified haemoglobin exceeded the reference range of teetotal controls in 50 % of the alcoholics but in only 24 % of social drinkers (Niemela and Israel, 1992). Modified haemoglobin could still be detected in samples from heavy drinkers who had abstained for up to 3 weeks. A similar elevation in modified haemoglobin was also observed by Lin coworkers (Lin et al., 1993).

Another, more analytical approach to the measurement of modified haemoglobin has also been used. The development of sensitive cation exchange liquid chromatographic methods (Sillanaukee and Koivula, 1990; Hazelett et al., 1993) has enabled this modified haemoglobin, often termed HbA1ach, to be studied in more detail. Further studies have shown that HbA1ach levels are elevated in the blood of alcoholics and heavy drinkers (> 280 g per week) when compared to controls. The level of HbA1ach also correlates with results from the Malmo-modified Michigan alcoholism screening test (Sillanaukee et al., 1991), again suggesting that measurement of HbA1ach may be a good marker of heavy alcohol intake. Another study has now shown that HbA1ach levels correlate with serum transaminase and CDT levels (Wickramasinghe et al., 1994), and that measurement by ELISA or chromatographically yield similar data (Sillanaukee et al., 1992). Analysis of modified haemoglobin from alcoholics has revealed that the likely sites of modification are the N-termini of the α- and β-globin chains (Gross et al., 1992), as well as unspecified internal residues (Gross et al., 1994). Chromatographic techniques with higher resolution are now suggesting that acetaldehyde-modified haemoglobin exists as at least three species (Chen et al., 1995; Itala et al., 1995; Hurme et al., 1998), each of which appears to be related to alcohol consumption. Finally, another study has shown that the measurement of modified haemoglobin is not affected by gender, drug misuse or degree of liver damage (Hazelett et al., 1998). Thus, there are many studies showing that acetaldehyde-modified haemoglobin has the potential to be a useful marker for alcohol abuse. However, there are some studies which suggest that conventional markers may be more useful under certain circumstances (Conduah Birt et al., 1998; Sarkola et al., 2000).

Little work has been done on the measurement of proteins modified by other metabolites of ethanol in samples from alcoholics.

Evidence for an immune response against modified proteins

There is a now a fairly extensive literature to show that proteins modified by reactive metabolites act as neoantigens to elicit an immune response against the modification (adduct; hapten) and against the carrier protein. However, although research has largely been limited to the detection of antibodies reactive with adducts, there are reports by one group of a cellular immune response against acetaldehyde-modified proteins (Terabayashi and Kolber, 1990; Kolber and Terabayashi, 1991). Many studies have now shown that rodents fed ethanol and human alcoholics generate antibodies reactive with proteins modified by ethanol metabolites in vitro. In 1986, Israel and coworkers were the first to demonstrate the production of anti-acetaldehyde adduct antibodies by animals (mice) chronically oxidizing ethanol. In a later study we demonstrated that the magnitude of this response was related to the time that the animals were fed ethanol (Worrall et al., 1989). In that study rats fed ethanol in their drinking water for 3 weeks were found to have a slight response against acetaldehyde adducts. At 3 months a much stronger response was observed, and at 27 months the maximal response was achieved. Thus, the magnitude of the immune response against the modified proteins appeared to be related to the cumulative ethanol dose. A further study revealed that antibodies reactive with at least two different classes of modification were generated in these animals (Worrall et al., 1994). Similar studies have demonstrated the generation of antibodies against proteins modified by α-hydroxyethyl radicals (Albano et al., 1996; Worrall et al., 2000), malondialdehyde (Worrall et al., 2000) and 4-hydroxynonenal (Tsukamoto et al., 1995). We have recently shown that rats fed the ethanol-containing form of the Lieber-DeCarli liquid diet for 10 weeks generated elevated immunoreactivity with proteins modified by indirect and direct ethanol metabolites when compared to their pair-fed controls (Worrall et al., 2000). Furthermore, they also produced higher concentrations of modified proteins than the control animals. Thus, at least for rats, measurement of either the modified proteins, or the antibodies reactive with them, can be used as a marker of alcohol intake. The picture is not so clear in humans.

There is a now a considerable body of evidence relating to the production of antibodies against epitopes derived from ethanol metabolites. Initial studies were carried out on antibodies reactive with acetaldehyde-derived modifications. Thus, several groups were able to detect antibodies reactive against acetaldehyde-modified proteins before they could demonstrate the presence of the modified proteins per se (Niemela et al., 1987; Hoerner et al., 1988; Worrall et al., 1989). These studies used ELISAs to measure reactivity of antibodies in plasma or serum with proteins modified by acetaldehyde in vitro. The conditions used to modify the proteins for use in the assays varied widely, making it possible that different modifications were being made to the proteins, and therefore different types of antibody were being detected in each study. I will discuss this further in the final section of this chapter. In rodent experiments there was a clear distinction between animals fed ethanol and their ethanol-naïve controls. In those experiments any animal with a high immunoreactivity against acetaldehyde-modified proteins could be definitively identified as an "alcoholic". This was not so in the human studies as high immunoreactivity was observed in some social drinkers (< 50 g ethanol per week for males and < 30 g per week for females) and in some teetotalers (Worrall et al., 1990). However, more individuals with high immunoreactivity were observed in the alcoholic groups in all of the studies (Niemela et al., 1987; Hoerner et al., 1988; Worrall et al., 1990).

At present most interest on antibody reactivity has focused on their interaction with modified proteins. It should however be noted that antibodies generated against modified proteins will also react with modified lipids. Studies by Trudell and coworkers (Trudell et al., 1990; 1991) have shown that antibodies raised against acetaldehyde-modified albumin will also react with acetaldehyde-modified dioleoyl phosphatidylethanolamine, presumably because the modification in both cases is of a similar nature. Thus, while it is possible that modified lipids are at least in part responsible for the generation of the anti-adduct antibodies, it is much easier to use modified proteins to detect and measure them. Furthermore, most of the research effort has been focused on the reactivity of antibodies with the chemically-derived modifications rather than looking at the reactivity with the carrier protein. Once a protein is modified the immune system generates antibodies against the carrier protein per se and the chemical modification. In an early study (Worrall et al., 1990) we noted that immunoreactivity with unmodified proteins was higher in alcoholics than in patients with non-alcoholic liver disease or social drinkers. There is also a potential for antibodies to be raised against an epitope which consists of part of the protein and the modification. There is some evidence to suggest this actually occurs. Koskinas and coworkers (Koskinas et al., 1992) demonstrated that antibodies from 70 % of patients with alcoholic hepatitis reacted with a 200 kDa cytosolic protein when it is was modified in vitro by acetaldehyde and then treated with a reducing agent. Similar antibodies could only be seen in 25 % of controls and 35 % of patients with non-alcoholic liver disease. The antibodies detected in this study must have a degree of carrier protein specificity since they only detected the 200 kDa protein even when other modified proteins were present. However, they did not recognise the 200 kDa protein when it was unmodified, suggesting that the epitope they reacted with was in large part due to the process of modification. These findings warrant further investigation.

Can antibodies reactive with proteins modified by ethanol metabolites be used as a marker of alcohol intake?

The initial results presented above prompted us to characterise the immune response against acetaldehyde adducts in more detail. To do this we decided to refine the ELISA we had previously used by modifying it so that we could detect different classes of immunoglobulins (IgG, IgA & IgM). Our previous study (Worrall et al., 1990) had used reagents that could only measure "total" immunoreactivity (i.e. the summation of all the classes of immunoglobulin). The rationale behind this decision to further characterize the immune response was that there were several reports of abnormalities in the composition of circulating immunoglobulins in alcoholics, especially those with liver disease. For example, significantly elevated levels of serum IgA have been observed in patients with alcoholic liver disease (van de Wiel et al., 1988). Furthermore, a characteristic "continuous" pattern of perisinusoidal IgA deposition was noticed in the livers of those individuals (Kater et al., 1979; Swerdlow et al., 1982; Swerdlow and Chowdhury,

1983; Amano et al., 1988). Antibodies of the IgA class that are reactive with liver plasma membranes in vitro have been isolated from alcoholic plasma (Burt et al., 1982). It is believed that the deposition of IgA may provide a chemotactic stimulus for neutrophils, the major inflammatory cells in alcoholic hepatitis, leading to localised tissue damage. The mechanisms behind the elevation of plasma IgA are unclear but it has been suggested that it may be due to damage of the gastric and intestinal mucosa such that IgA-secreting mucosal plasma cells become over stimulated and produce more IgA (Kater et al., 1979). In addition, peripheral blood mononuclear cells may spontaneously produce IgA (van de Wiel et al., 1987). These increases in production may also be linked to a decrease in catabolism (Delacroix et al., 1983) that may be related to a decrease in the ability of the liver to remove IgA from the circulation (Brown and Kloppel, 1989). The deposition of IgA in the liver is unlikely to be a non-specific mechanism as other diseases such is IgA myeloma, which are also characterized by high plasma IgA levels, do not show this pattern of hepatic IgA deposition. A much more likely explanation is that deposition occurs due to a specific interaction between the antibodies and ethanol-induced epitopes in the liver. Another characteristic of alcoholism, and of alcoholic liver disease, is the presence of circulating immune complexes derived from IgA and ethanol-induced antigens (Kanagasundaram et al., 1977; Coppo et al., 1985). Normally immune complexes are efficiently removed from the circulation and their presence in alcoholics suggests decreased clearance, again potentially due to decreased liver function. From this evidence we thought it would be interesting to look at IgA reactivity with acetaldehyde-modified proteins in alcoholics.

Our first study (Worrall et al., 1991a) showed that alcoholics, patients with non-alcoholic liver disease and social drinkers exhibited a large IgM response to acetaldehyde-modified proteins but did not generate a significant IgG response. Thus, measurement of IgM or IgG reactivity against acetaldehyde-modified epitopes was not useful in detecting alcohol abuse. However, alcoholics did express a significantly higher IgA response than either of the other two groups. The magnitude of the IgA response was not related to the stage of alcoholic liver disease, appearing to be related to excessive alcohol intake instead. Thus, measurement of IgA reactivity had potential as a marker for excessive alcohol intake. Our second study (Worrall et al., 1996) was designed to determine whether there was a linear relationship between the amount of alcohol consumed and the magnitude of the IgA response. To do this we analysed samples from three groups of individuals with differing alcohol intake

(1) social drinkers (< 30 g ethanol per week for females and < 50 g per week for males);
(2) heavy drinkers (> 130 but < 540 g ethanol per week for females and > 150 but < 1000 g per week for males); and
(3) (> 800 g ethanol per week for females and > 1000 g per week for males).

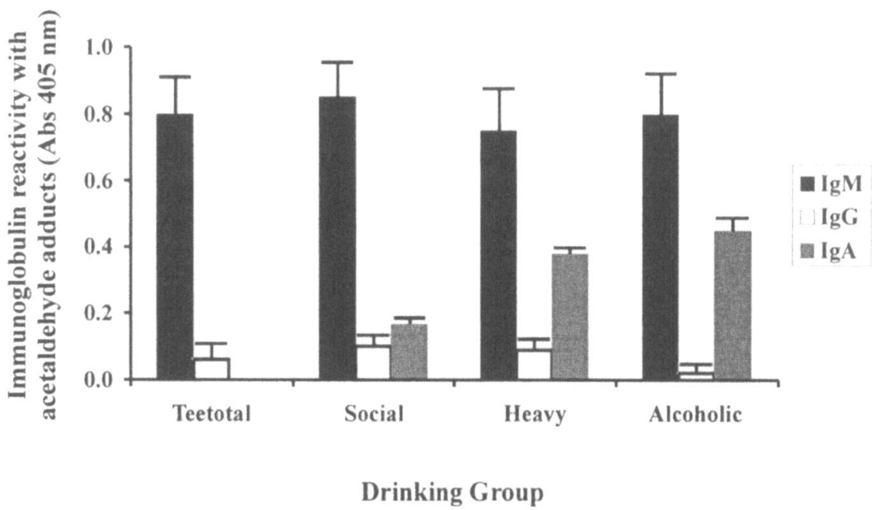

Figure 2 The reactivity of various classes of immunoglobulin with haemoglobin modified by acetaldehyde in vitro.

(Data are taken from Worrall et al. (1996) and are presented as mean ± SEM)

This study showed that IgA immunoreactivity had a moderate correlation with self-reported alcohol intake, which may not be a totally true reflection of the actual amount of ethanol consumed. There were three other interesting pieces of data to come out of this study. The first was that teetotalers do not produce IgA immunoreactivity with acetaldehyde-derived epitopes, suggesting that IgA reactivity against acetaldehyde-modified epitopes is related solely to alcohol intake. The second was that teetotalers do express IgM reactivity against the modified epitopes suggesting that this response might not be related to alcohol intake. The final interesting data was that the magnitude of the IgA response was not related to the amount of acetaldehyde-modified albumin present in the circulation. This was somewhat surprising since it is likely that modified plasma proteins are some of the antigens which would induce the production of the antibodies. However, it is possible that there may not be a linear correlation between the amount of antibody produced and the amount of antigen present. Alternatively it is possible that the modified albumin is not one of the antigens which generated the antibodies we measured. Our third study (Worrall et al., 1998) compared the measurement of IgA immunoreactivity with acetaldehyde-modified proteins with the presently used markers of alcohol abuse (Figure 3). In this study IgA immunoreactivity did not correlate with conventional markers of alcohol abuse such as mean corpuscular volume or plasma γ-glutamyl transferase or transaminase (alanine and aspartate) activities. However, while there was a weak correlation between IgA immunoreactivity and CDT levels, there were many individuals that did not exceed the normal range for both. For example, in the male alcoholic group 97 % of the individuals exceeded the normal range for either IgA reactivity or for CDT levels, only 57 % of the individuals exceeded the normal range for both. This suggests that the concurrent use of CDT and IgA reactivity may lead to better identification of high alcohol intake. Similar results have been obtained in another study (Viitala et al., 1997) which showed that IgA reactivity correlated with serum bilirubin and IL-6 levels. They were also able to detect substantial IgG reactivity in 42 % of patients with alcoholic liver disease and show that it correlated with inflammation and necrosis. Significant IgA or IgG reactivity was only seen in 4 % of healthy controls. The only major discrepancy between the two studies was that the second one was unable to detect any IgM reactivity with acetaldehyde modifications.

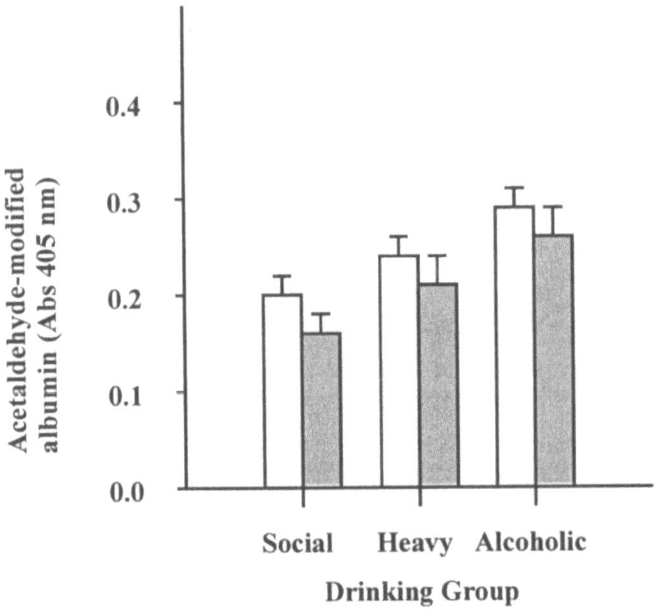

Figure 3 Acetaldehyde-modified albumin as measured by ELISA in groups with varying alcohol intake

(Data are taken from Worrall et al. (1998) and are presented as mean ± SEM. Open bars represent females and shaded bars represent males.)

Again when looking at the measurement of antibodies against proteins modified as a result of alcohol metabolism the main research effort has been on those modified by acetaldehyde. This is not surprising as acetaldehyde is by far the most abundant species produced, having approximate molar equivalency with the amount of ethanol consumed. However, antibodies against α-hydroxyethyl radical- and malondialdehyde-modified proteins have been detected in human alcoholics. The effect of alcohol consumption on the plasma concentrations of malondialdehyde and antibodies directed against malondialdehyde adducts on proteins has been investigated in supposedly healthy men who consumed only low or moderate amounts of alcohol and in alcoholic patients without severe liver disease (Lecomte et al., 1994). Plasma concentrations of malondialdehyde, and antibodies reactive with malondialdehyde-modified proteins, were higher in the alcoholics when compared to controls. In the alcoholic group, three weeks after cessation of drinking, plasma concentrations of malondialdehyde and the titre of antibodies were decreased. In another study higher titres of antibodies reactive with malondialdehyde-modified protein were observed in alcoholics but the elevation was not statistically significant when compared to controls (Chancerelle et al., 1998). In a recent study of alcoholics, heavy drinkers and social drinking controls significantly higher IgG immunoreactivity with MAA 2:1 was observed (Rolla et al., 2000). Alcoholics with hepatitis or cirrhosis expressed the highest immunoreactivity whereas patients with non-alcoholic liver disease had much lower levels. These data suggest that measurement of IgG immunoreactivity with MAA 2:1 adducts may be a good marker for alcoholic liver damage but not alcohol intake per se.

Problems and future directions

The measurement of both ethanol metabolite-modified proteins and their associated antibodies has shown promise in the development of new markers of alcohol intake. However, there is one major problem which has so far clouded previous results and is holding up future work. That problem is the chemical nature of the modifications formed in vivo and in vitro. Without an understanding of the nature of the adducts formed during modification procedures used to prepare modified proteins in vitro it is impossible to know what is being measured by the reagents generated from their use. For example, if the modified protein is used to generate antibodies, the exact reactivity of the antibodies is unknown. The situation is no better if the modified protein is used as the coating antigen for an ELISA as the immunoreactivity measured is then largely undefined. To rectify this situation we and others are undertaking studies to chemically define the adducts produced under various conditions (Thiele et al., 1994; Fowles et al., 1996; Tuma et al., 1996; Graham et al., 1998). Production of defined adducts has allowed the generation of some antibodies with known reactivity, enabling measurement of specific adducts to be carried out (Worrall et al., 2000; Rolla et al., 2000). Such antibodies so far generated include those with reactivity with N-ethylated amino groups (Thiele et al., 1994) or those with reactivity against the MAA 2:1 adduct (Tuma et al., 1996).

Reagents with known chemical structure or immunoreactivity will revolutionise this area of research and herald an explosive expansion of our understanding. The prospects are bright that, in the next few years, research in this area will generate a highly specific biological marker for chronic alcohol intake.

Acknowledgments

The author wishes to thank his long-term collaborators Peter Wilce and John de Jersey for their friendship, advice and support over the last thirteen years. I also wish to thank Dean Tuma and Geoff Thiele for their generous gifts of polyclonal antisera and monoclonal antibodies against chemically-defined adducts, and for their support and friendship. I look forward to further collaborations with them.

References

Albano, E., Tomasi, A., Goria Gatti, L. and Dianzani, M. U. (1988) Spin trapping of free radical species produced during the microsomal metabolism of ethanol. Chem Biol Interact 65, 223-34.

Albano, E., Clot, P., Morimoto, M., Tomasi, A., Ingelman Sundberg, M. and French, S. W. (1996) Role of cytochrome P4502E1-dependent formation of hydroxyethyl free radical in the development of liver damage in rats intragastrically fed with ethanol. Hepatology 23, 155-63.

Amano, K., Tsukada, K., Takeuchi, T., Fukuda, Y. and Nagura, H. (1988) IgA deposition in alcoholic liver disease. Am J Clin Pathol 89, 728-734.

Baraona, E., Di Padova, C., Tabasco, J. and Lieber, C. S. (1987a) Red blood cells: a new major modality for acetaldehyde transport from liver to other tissues. Life Sci 40, 253-8.

Baraona, E., DiPadova, C., Tabasco, J. and Lieber, C. S. (1987 b) Transport of acetaldehyde in red blood cells. Alcohol Alcohol Suppl 1, 203-6.

Behrens, U. J., Hoerner, M., Lasker, J. M. and Lieber, C. S. (1988) Formation of acetaldehyde adducts with ethanol-inducible P450IIE1 in vivo. Biochem Biophys Res Commun 154, 584-90.

Brown, W. R. and Kloppel, T. M. (1989) The liver and IgA: immunological, cell biological and clinical implications. Hepatology 9, 763-784.

Burt, A. D., Anthony, R. S., Hislop, W. S., Bouchier, I. A. and MacSween, R. N. (1982) Liver membrane antibodies in alcoholic liver disease: 1. prevalence and immunoglobulin class. Gut 23, 221-5.

Chancerelle, Y., Mathieu, J. and Kergonou, J. F. (1998) Antibodies against malondialdehyde-modified proteins. Induction and ELISA measurement of specific antibodies. Methods Mol Biol 108, 111-8.

Chen, H. M., Scott, B. K., Braun, K. P. and Peterson, C. M. (1995) Validated fluorimetric HPLC analysis of acetaldehyde in hemoglobin fractions separated by cation exchange chromatography: three new peaks associated with acetaldehyde. Alcohol Clin Exp Res 19, 939-44.

Clot, P., Tabone, M., Arico, S. and Albano, E. (1994) Monitoring oxidative damage in patients with liver cirrhosis and different daily alcohol intake. Gut 35, 1637-43.

Clot, P., Albano, E., Eliasson, E., Tabone, M., Arico, S., Israel, Y., Moncada, C. and Ingelman Sundberg, M. (1996) Cytochrome P4502E1 hydroxyethyl radical adducts as the major antigen in autoantibody formation among alcoholics. Gastroenterology 111, 206-16.

Collins, D. J. and Lapsley, H. M. (1996) estimating the economic costs of drug abuse in Australia in 1988 and 1992. Commonwealth of australia Department of Health and Aging Monograph Series, No. 30.

Conduah Birt, J. E., Shuker, D. E. and Farmer, P. B. (1998) Stable acetaldehyde--protein adducts as biomarkers of alcohol exposure. Chem Res Toxicol 11, 136-42.

Coppo, R., Arico, S., Basolo, B., Roccattelo, D., Amore, A., Tabone, M., De la Pierre, M., Sessa, A., Delacroix, D. L. and Vaerman, J. P. (1985) Presence and origin of IgA1- and IgA2-containing circulating immune complexes in alcoholic liver diseases with and without glomerulonephritis. Clin Immunol Immunopathol 35, 1-8.

Delacroix, D. L., Elkon, K. B., Geubel, A. P., Hodgson, H. F., Dive, C. and Vaerman, J. P. (1983) Changes in size, subclass and metabolic properties of serum immunoglobulin A in liver diseases and other diseases with high serum immunoglobulin A. Am J Clin Invest 71, 358-367.

Donohue, T. M., Jr., Tuma, D. J. and Sorrell, M. F. (1983) Binding of metabolically derived acetaldehyde to hepatic proteins in vitro. Lab Invest 49, 226-9.

Esterbauer, H., Schaur, R. J. and Zollner, H. (1991) Chemistry and biochemistry of 4-hydroxynonenal, malonaldehyde and related aldehydes. Free Radic Biol Med 11, 81-128.

Fowles, L. F., Beck, E., Worrall, S., Shanley, B. C. and de Jersey, J. (1996) The formation and stability of imidazolidinone adducts from acetaldehyde and model peptides. A kinetic study with implications for protein modification in alcohol abuse. Biochem Pharmacol 51, 1259-67.

Graham, V., Worrall, S. and de Jersey, J. (1998) Analysis of adducts formed between acetaldehyde and thiol-containing peptides. Paper presented at the Ninth congress of the International Society for Biomedical research on Alcoholism, Copenhagen, Denmark, 1998. Alcohol Clin Exp Res 22 Suppl 3, 174A.

Gross, M. D., Gapstur, S. M., Belcher, J. D., Scanlan, G. and Potter, J. D. (1992) The identification and partial characterization of acetaldehyde adducts of hemoglobin occurring in vivo: a possible marker of alcohol consumption. Alcohol Clin Exp Res 16, 1093-103.

Gross, M. D., Hays, R., Gapstur, S. M., Chaussee, M. and Potter, J. D. (1994) Evidence for the formation of multiple types of acetaldehyde-haemoglobin adducts. Alcohol Alcohol 29, 31-41.
Hazelett, S. E., Liebelt, R. A. and Truitt, E. B., Jr. (1993) Improved separation of acetaldehyde-induced hemoglobin. Alcohol Clin Exp Res 17, 1107-11.
Hazelett, S. E., Liebelt, R. A., Brown, W. J., Androulakakis, V., Jarjoura, D. and Truitt, E. B., Jr. (1998) Evaluation of acetaldehyde-modified hemoglobin and other markers of chronic heavy alcohol use: effects of gender and hemoglobin concentration. Alcohol Clin Exp Res 22, 1813-9.
Hoerner, M., Behrens, U. J., Worner, T. M., Blacksberg, I., Braly, L. F., Schaffner, F. and Lieber, C. S. (1988) The role of alcoholism and liver disease in the appearance of serum antibodies against acetaldehyde adducts. Hepatology 8, 569-574.
Holstege, A., Bedossa, P., Poynard, T., Kollinger, M., Chaput, J. C., Houglum, K. and Chojkier, M. (1994) Acetaldehyde-modified epitopes in liver biopsy specimens of alcoholic and nonalcoholic patients: localization and association with progression of liver fibrosis. Hepatology 19, 367-74. [published erratum appears in Hepatology 1994 Dec;20(6):1664].
Houglum, K., Filip, M., Witztum, J. L. and Chojkier, M. (1990) Malondialdehyde and 4-hydroxynonenal protein adducts in plasma and liver of rats with iron overload. J Clin Invest 86, 1991-8.
Hurme, L., Seppa, K., Rajaniemi, H. and Sillanaukee, P. (1998) Chromatographically identified alcohol-induced haemoglobin adducts as markers of alcohol abuse among women. Eur J Clin Invest 28, 87-94.
Iimuro, Y., Bradford, B. U., Gao, W., Kadiiska, M., Mason, R. P., Stefanovic, B., Brenner, D. A. and Thurman, R. G. (1996) Detection of alpha-hydroxyethyl free radical adducts in the pancreas after chronic exposure to alcohol in the rat. Mol Pharmacol 50, 656-61.
Itala, L., Seppa, K., Turpeinen, U. and Sillanaukee, P. (1995) Separation of hemoglobin acetaldehyde adducts by high-performance liquid chromatography-cation-exchange chromatography. Anal Biochem 224, 323-9.
Kamimura, S., Gaal, K., Britton, R. S., Bacon, B. R., Triadafilopoulos, G. and Tsukamoto, H. (1992) Increased 4-hydroxynonenal levels in experimental alcoholic liver disease: association of lipid peroxidation with liver fibrogenesis. Hepatology 16, 448-53.
Kanagasundaram, N., Kakumu, S., Chen, T. and Leevy, C. M. (1977) Alcohol hyalin antigen (AHAg) and antibody (AHAb) in alcoholic hepatitis. Gastroenterology 73, 1368-1373.
Kater, L., Jobsis, A. C., Baart de la Faille-Kuyper, E. H., Vogten, A. J. M. and Grijm, R. (1979) Alcoholic hepatic disease: specificity of IgA deposits in the liver. Am J Pathol 71, 51-7.
Kearley, M. L., Patel, A., Chien, J. and Tuma, D. J. (1999) Observation of a new nonfluorescent malondialdehyde-acetaldehyde-protein adduct by 13C NMR spectroscopy. Chem Res Toxicol 12, 100-5.
Kolber, M. A. and Terabayashi, H. (1991) Cytotoxic T lymphocytes can be generated against acetaldehyde-modified syngeneic cells. Alcohol Alcohol Suppl 1, 277-80.
Koskinas, J., Kenna, J. G., Bird, G. L., Alexander, G. J. and Williams, R. (1992) Immunoglobulin A antibody to a 200-kilodalton cytosolic acetaldehyde adduct in alcoholic hepatitis. Gastroenterology 103, 1860-7.
Lecomte, E., Herbeth, B., Pirollet, P., Chancerelle, Y., Arnaud, J., Musse, N., Paille, F., Siest, G. and Artur, Y. (1994) Effect of alcohol consumption on blood antioxidant nutrients and oxidative stress indicators. Am J Clin Nutr 60, 255-61.
Li, C. J., Nanji, A. A., Siakotos, A. N. and Lin, R. C. (1997) Acetaldehyde-modified and 4-hydroxynonenal-modified proteins in the livers of rats with alcoholic liver disease. Hepatology 26, 650-7.
Lieber, C. S. (1999) Microsomal ethanol-oxidizing system (MEOS): the first 30 years (1968-1998): a review. Alcohol Clin Exp Res 23, 991-1007.
Lieber, C. S. (2000) Ethnic and gender differences in ethanol metabolism. Alcohol Clin Exp Res 24, 417-8.
Lin, R. C., Smith, R. S. and Lumeng, L. (1988) Detection of a protein-acetaldehyde adduct in the liver of rats fed alcohol chronically. J Clin Invest 81, 615-9.
Lin, R. C., Lumeng, L., Shahidi, S., Kelly, T. and Pound, D. C. (1990) Protein-acetaldehyde adducts in serum of alcoholic patients. Alcohol Clin Exp Res 14, 438-43.
Lin, R. C., Shahidi, S., Kelly, T. J., Lumeng, C. and Lumeng, L. (1993) Measurement of hemoglobin-acetaldehyde adduct in alcoholic patients. Alcohol Clin Exp Res 17, 669-74.
Medina, V. A., Donohue, T. M., Jr., Sorrell, M. F. and Tuma, D. J. (1985) Covalent binding of acetaldehyde to hepatic proteins during ethanol oxidation. J-Lab-Clin-Med 105, 5-10.

Nicholls, R., de Jersey, J., Worrall, S. and Wilce, P. (1992) Modification of proteins and other biological molecules by acetaldehyde: adduct structure and functional significance. Int J Biochem 24, 1899-906.

Nicholls, R. M., Fowles, L. F., Worrall, S., de Jersey, J. and Wilce, P. A. (1994) Distribution and turnover of acetaldehyde-modified proteins in liver and blood of ethanol-fed rats. Alcohol Alcohol 29, 149-57.

Niemela, O., Klajner, F., Orrego, H., Vidins, E., Blendis, L. and Israel, Y. (1987) Antibodies against acetaldehyde-modified protein epitopes in human alcoholics. Hepatology 7, 1210-4.

Niemela, O., Israel, Y., Mizoi, Y., Fukunaga, T. and Eriksson, C. J. (1990) Hemoglobin-acetaldehyde adducts in human volunteers following acute ethanol ingestion. Alcohol Clin Exp Res 14, 838-41.

Niemela, O., Halmesmaki, E. and Ylikorkala, O. (1991a) Hemoglobin-acetaldehyde adducts are elevated in women carrying alcohol-damaged fetuses. Alcohol-Clin-Exp-Res 15, 1007-10.

Niemela, O., Juvonen, T. and Parkkila, S. (1991 b) Immunohistochemical demonstration of acetaldehyde-modified epitopes in human liver after alcohol consumption. J Clin Invest 87, 1367-74.

Niemela, O. and Israel, Y. (1992) Hemoglobin-acetaldehyde adducts in human alcohol abusers. Lab Invest 67, 246-52.

Niemela, O., Parkkila, S., Yla Herttuala, S., Villanueva, J., Ruebner, B. and Halsted, C. H. (1995) Sequential acetaldehyde production, lipid peroxidation, and fibrogenesis in micropig model of alcohol-induced liver disease. Hepatology 22, 1208-14.

Niemela, O., Parkkila, S., Pasanen, M., Iimur, Y., Bradford, B. and Thurman, R. G. (1998) Early alcoholic liver injury: formation of protein adducts with acetaldehyde and lipid peroxidation products, and expression of CYP2E1 and CYP3A. Alcohol-Clin-Exp-Res 22, 2118-24.

Ohhira, M., Ohtake, T., Matsumoto, A., Saito, H., Ikuta, K., Fujimoto, Y., Ono, M., Toyokuni, S. and Kohgo, Y. (1998) Immunohistochemical detection of 4-hydroxy-2-nonenal-modified-protein adducts in human alcoholic liver diseases. Alcohol Clin Exp Res 22, 145s-149s.

Paradis, V., Mathurin, P., Ratziu, V., Poynard, T. and Bedossa, P. (1996) Binding of apolipoprotein A-I and acetaldehyde-modified apolipoprotein A-I to liver extracellular matrix. Hepatology 23, 1232-8.

Rolla, R., Vay, D., Mottaran, E., Parodi, M., Traverso, N., Arico, S., Sartori, M., Bellomo, G., Klassen, L. W., Thiele, G. M., Tuma, D. J. and Albano, E. (2000) Detection of circulating antibodies against malondialdehyde-acetaldehyde adducts in patients with alcohol-induced liver disease. Hepatology 31, 878-84.

San George, R. C. and Hoberman, H. D. (1986) Reaction of acetaldehyde with hemoglobin. J Biol Chem 261, 6811-21.

Sarkola, T., Eriksson, C. J., Niemela, O., Sillanaukee, P. and Halmesmaki, E. (2000) Mean cell volume and gamma-glutamyl transferase are superior to carbohydrate-deficient transferrin and hemoglobin-acetaldehyde adducts in the follow-up of pregnant women with alcohol abuse. Acta-Obstet-Gynecol-Scand 79, 359-66.

Sillanaukee, P. and Koivula, T. (1990) Detection of a new acetaldehyde-induced hemoglobin fraction HbA1ach by cation exchange liquid chromatography. Alcohol Clin Exp Res 14, 842-6.

Sillanaukee, P., Seppa, K. and Koivula, T. (1991) Association of a haemoglobin-acetaldehyde adduct with questionnaire results on heavy drinkers. Alcohol Alcohol 26, 519-25.

Sillanaukee, P., Seppa, K., Koivula, T., Israel, Y. and Niemela, O. (1992) Acetaldehyde-modified hemoglobin as a marker of alcohol consumption: comparison of two new methods. J-Lab-Clin-Med 120, 42-7.

Stibler, H. and Hultcrantz, R. (1987) Carbohydrate-deficient transferrin in serum in patients with liver diseases. Alcohol Clin Exp Res 11, 468-73.

Stockham, T. L. and Blanke, R. V. (1988) Investigation of an acetaldehyde-hemoglobin adduct in alcoholics. Alcohol Clin Exp Res 12, 748-54.

Swerdlow, M. A., Chowdhury, L. N. and Horn, T. (1982) Patterns of IgA deposition in liver tissues in alcoholic liver disease. Am J Clin Pathol 77, 259-66.

Swerdlow, M. A. and Chowdhury, L. N. (1983) IgA subclasses in liver tissues in alcoholic liver disease. Am J Clin Pathol 80, 283-9.

Terabayashi, H. and Kolber, M. A. (1990) The generation of cytotoxic T lymphocytes against acetaldehyde-modified syngeneic cells. Alcohol Clin Exp Res 14, 893-9.

Thiele, G. M., Wegter, K. M., Sorrell, M. F., Tuma, D. J., McDonald, T. L. and Klassen, L. W. (1994) Specificity of N-ethyl lysine of a monoclonal antibody to acetaldehyde-modified proteins prepared under reducing conditions. Biochem Pharmacol 48, 183-9.

Thiele, G. M., Tuma, D. J., Willis, M. S., Miller, J. A., McDonald, T. L., Sorrell, M. F. and Klassen, L. W. (1998) Soluble proteins modified with acetaldehyde and malondialdehyde are immunogenic in the absence of adjuvant. Alcohol Clin Exp Res 22, 1731-9.

Trudell, J. R., Ardies, C. M. and Anderson, W. R. (1990) Cross-reactivity of antibodies raised against acetaldehyde adducts of protein with acetaldehyde adducts of phosphatidyl-ethanolamine: possible role in alcoholic cirrhosis. Mol Pharmacol 38, 587-93.

Trudell, J. R., Ardies, C. M., Green, C. E. and Allen, K. (1991) Binding of anti-acetaldehyde IgG antibodies to hepatocytes with an acetaldehyde-phosphatidylethanolamine adduct on their surface. Alcohol Clin Exp Res 15, 295-9.

Tsukamoto, H., Horne, W., Kamimura, S., Niemela, O., Parkkila, S., Yla Herttuala, S. and Brittenham, G. M. (1995) Experimental liver cirrhosis induced by alcohol and iron. J Clin Invest 96, 620-30.

Tuma, D. J. and Sorrell, M. F. (1995) The role of acetaldehyde adducts in liver injury. In Alcoholic Liver Disease: Pathology and Pathogenesis., Hall, P. ed, pp. 89-99. Edward Arnold, London.

Tuma, D. J., Thiele, G. M., Xu, D., Klassen, L. W. and Sorrell, M. F. (1996) Acetaldehyde and malondialdehyde react together to generate distinct protein adducts in the liver during long-term ethanol administration. Hepatology 23, 872-80.

Tuma, D. J., Kearley, M. L., Worrall, S. and Thiele, G. M. (2001) Elucidation of a reaction scheme describing malon dialdehyde-acetaldehyde-protein adduct formation. Chem Res Toxicol, in press.

Van de Wiel, A., Delacroix, D. L., van Hattum, J., Schuurman, H. J. and Kater, L. (1987) Characteristics of serum IgA and liver IgA deposits in alcoholic liver disease. Hepatology 7, 95-9.

Van de Wiel, A., van Hattum, J., Schuurman, H. J. and Kater, L. (1988) Immunoglobulin A in the diagnosis of alcoholic liver disease. Gastroenterology 94, 457-62.

Viitala, K., Israel, Y., Blake, J. E. and Niemela, O. (1997) Serum IgA, IgG, and IgM antibodies directed against acetaldehyde-derived epitopes: relationship to liver disease severity and alcohol consumption. Hepatology 25, 1418-24.

Wickramasinghe, S. N., Corridan, B., Hasan, R. and Marjot, D. H. (1994) Correlations between acetaldehyde-modified haemoglobin, carbohydrate-deficient transferrin (CDT) and haematological abnormalities in chronic alcoholism. Alcohol Alcohol 29, 415-23.

Worrall, S., de Jersey, J., Shanley, B. C. and Wilce, P. A. (1989) Ethanol induces the production of antibodics to acetaldehyde-modified epitopes in rats. Alcohol Alcohol 24, 217-23.

Worrall, S., de Jersey, J., Shanley, B. C. and Wilce, P. A. (1990) Antibodies against acetaldehyde-modified epitopes: presence in alcoholic, non-alcoholic liver disease and control subjects. Alcohol Alcohol 25, 509-17.

Worrall, S., de Jersey, J., Shanley, B. C. and Wilce, P. A. (1991a) Alcohol abusers exhibit a higher IgA response to acetaldehyde-modified proteins. Alcohol Alcohol Suppl 1, 261-4.

Worrall, S., de Jersey, J., Shanley, B. C. and Wilce, P. A. (1991 b) Detection of stable acetaldehyde-modified proteins in the livers of ethanol-fed rats. Alcohol Alcohol 26, 437-44.

Worrall, S., de Jersey, J., Shanley, B. C. and Wilce, P. A. (1994) Anti-acetaldehyde adduct antibodies generated by ethanol-fed rats react with reduced and unreduced acetaldehyde-modified proteins. Alcohol Alcohol 29, 43-50.

Worrall, S., de Jersey, J., Wilce, P. A., Seppa, K., Hurme, L. and Sillanaukee, P. (1996) Relationship between alcohol intake and immunoglobulin a immunoreactivity with acetaldehyde-modified bovine serum albumin. Alcohol Clin Exp Res 20, 836-40.

Worrall, S., de Jersey, J., Wilce, P. A., Seppa, K., Hurme, L. and Sillanaukee, P. (1998) Comparison of carbohydrate-deficient transferrin, immunoglobulin A antibodies reactive with acetaldehyde-modified protein and acetaldehyde-modified albumin with conventional markers of alcohol consumption. Alcohol Clin Exp Res 22, 1921-6.

Worrall, S., de Jersey, J. and Wilce, P. A. (2000) Comparison of the formation of proteins modified by direct and indirect ethanol metabolites in the liver and blood of rats fed the Lieber-DeCarli liquid diet. Alcohol Alcohol 35, 164-170.

Xu, D., Thiele, G. M., Kearley, M. L., Haugen, M. D., Klassen, L. W., Sorrell, M. F. and Tuma, D. J. (1997) Epitope characterization of malondialdehyde-acetaldehyde adducts using an enzyme-linked immunosorbent assay. Chem Res Toxicol 10, 978-86.

Yokoyama, H., Ishii, H., Nagata, S., Moriya, S., Ito, T., Kato, S. and Tsuchiya, M. (1993) Heterogeneity of hepatic acetaldehyde adducts in guinea-pigs after chronic ethanol administration: an immunohistochemical analysis with monoclonal and polyclonal antibodies against acetaldehyde-modified protein epitopes. Alcohol Alcohol Suppl 1a, 91-7.

Zhu, Y., Fillenwarth, M. J., Crabb, D., Lumeng, L. and Lin, R. C. (1996) Identification of the 37-kd rat liver protein that forms an acetaldehyde adduct in vivo as D^4-3-ketosteroid 5 β-reductase. Hepatology 23, 115-22.

Salsolinol - An endogenous neurotoxin in the biology of alcoholism

Frank Musshoff

Institute of Legal Medicine
Rheinische Friedrich-Wilhelms-University
Stiftsplatz 12
53111 Bonn
Germany

Abstract

Similarities between alcoholism and morphinism concerning the development of an addiction and symptoms of withdrawal led to the hypothesis that opiate-active compounds might be formed endogenously during the establishment of alcohol addiction. This theory was supported by the proof of the in vivo formation of simple tetrahydroisoquinoline alkaloids like salsolinol via Pictet-Spengler reaction from dopamine and the ethanol oxidation product acetaldehyde in the human body. Salsolinol was demonstrated to have a variety of neuropharmacological and cytotoxic effects and shows an affinity to the dopamine receptors. Definite evidence for a salsolinol formation in elevated concentrations after alcohol abuse is still lacking. In systematic regional studies using human brains we found significant amounts of salsolinol in the dopaminergic system, which is responsible for addiction processes. The possibility that biosynthesis of salsolinol occurs through a stereospecific enzymatic reaction was considered and both salsolinol enantiomers were found in human brain samples with no correlations between levels of salsolinol and dopamine. These findings do not support the hypothesis that only an enantio-selective synthesis of (R)-salsolinol by a putative salsolinol synthase is responsible for the in vivo formation.

1. Introduction

Similarities between alcoholism and morphinism concerning the production of dependence and symptoms of withdrawal led to the hypothesis that opiate-active compounds might be formed endogenously during the establishment of alcohol addiction (Cohen and Collins, 1970; Davis and Walsh, 1970). This theory was supported by the proof of the in vivo formation of various alkaloids in the human body. One hypothesis invoked the ethanol metabolite acetaldehyde as a critical intermediate in the biosynthesis of opiate-active compounds (Haber and Melzig, 1992). Acetaldehyde can condense directly with catecholamines in tissues to form substituted 6,7-dihydroxy-1,2,3,4-tetrahydroisoquinolines (TIQ). The most discussed compound is salsolinol (SAL; 1-methyl-6,7-dihydroy-1,2,3,4-tetrahydroisoquinoline). SAL might be formed in vivo by a non-enzymatic ring cyclization of dopamine with the ethanol oxidation product acetaldehyde to yield the racemic mixture of both enantiomers (Figure 1). Another pathway is the condensation of dopamine with pyruvic acid, followed by enzymatic decarboxylation and reduction (Robbins, 1968; Brossi, 1982). Additionally the formation of complex tetrahydroisochinoline alkaloids like tetrahydropapaveroline (THP) during alcohol consumption is assumed, which are discussed as connecting links between alcoholism and morphinism (Figure 2).

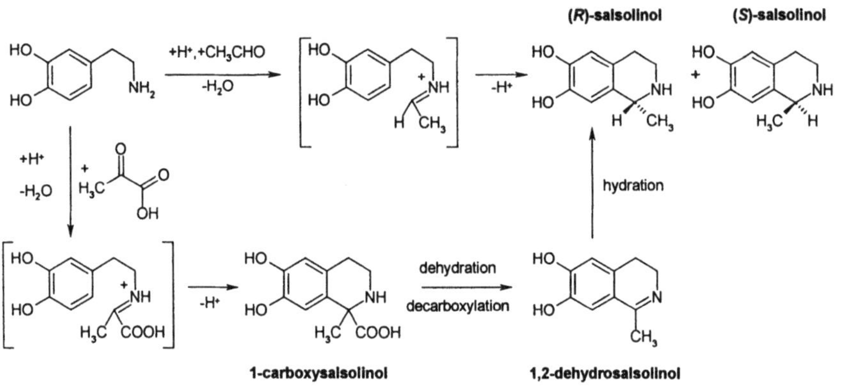

Figure 1 SAL might be formed in vivo by a non-enzymatic ring cyclization of dopamine (DA) with the ethanol oxidation product acetaldehyde to yield the racemic mixture of both enantiomers. Another pathway is the condensation of dopamine with pyruvic acid. SAL is formed from the intermediate 1-carboxysalsolinol via oxidative decarboxylation to 1,2-dihydrosalsolinol followed by hydration.

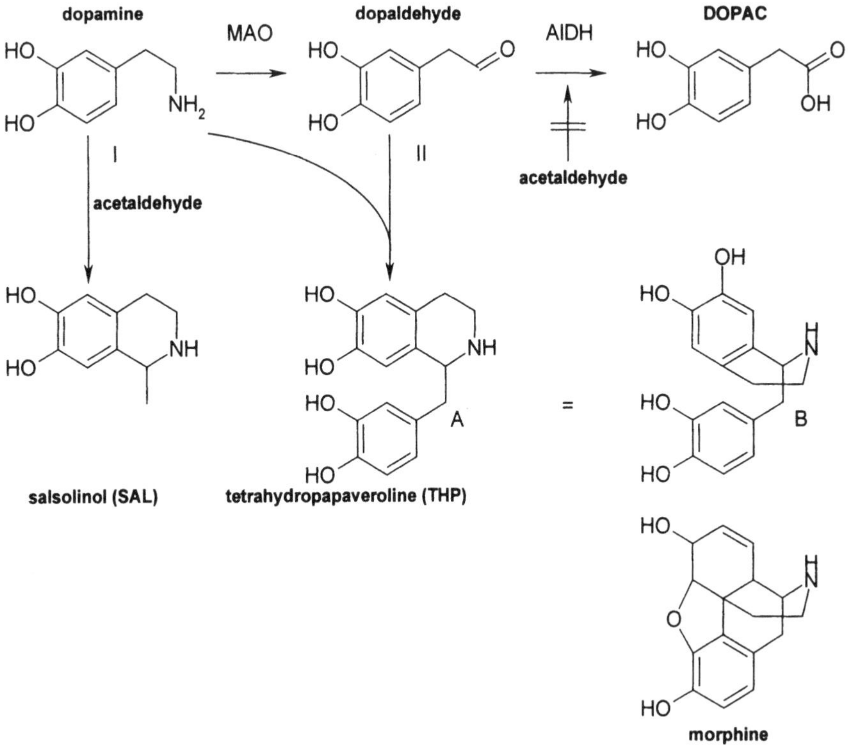

Figure 2 During alcohol consumption the aldehyde dehydrogenase (AlDH) is inhibited by the ethanol oxidation product acetaldehyde, and so dopaldehyde can condense with dopamine to form the complex alkaloid tetrahydropapaveroline (THP) (I). Additionally salsolinol is formed via Pictet-Spengler reaction from dopamine and acetaldehyde (II). THP is structural related to morphine (B). This is the reason for some groups to assume the possibility of secondary reactions of THP in the mammalian body to form pharmacological relevant alkaloids from the morphinan-, protoberberine- or apomorphine-type which are discussed as connecting links between alcoholism and morphinism. (MAO = monoamine oxidase; AlDH = aldehyde dehydrogenase; DOPAC = dihydroxyphenyl acetic acid).

Recently, it was suggested that (R)-SAL might be formed enzymatically by stereospecific condensation of dopamine with pyruvic acid (Naoi et al., 1995a). It has also been reported that N-methyldopamine (epinine) occurs in the human brain. Although the enzymatic N-methylation of SAL into N-methyl-salsolinol (NMSAL) was confirmed by in vivo microdialysis in the rat brain (Maruyama et al., 1992), an in vitro experiment suggested that it is also formed from epinine and acetaldehyde by Pictet-Spengler reaction (Kajita et al., 1994).

Norsalsolinol (NorSAL; 6,7-dihydroxy-1,2,3,4-tetrahydroisoquinoline) is formed non-enzymatically in vivo by Pictet-Spengler condensation of dopamine and formaldehyde. Formaldehyde is 15 times as reactive as acetaldehyde in the Pictet-Spengler reaction with dopamine. The level of NorSAL may be of interest in alcoholism, where, particularly during withdrawal, the levels of methanol, formaldehyde and formate increase significantly.

2. Salsolinol

2.1. Natural occurrence of salsolinol

TIQs are precursors of a wide array of alkaloids, e.g. protoberberine, papaverine, morphine, aporphine, thebaine, benzophenanthrene, and phthalideisoquinoline classes. Salsoline was the first TIQ isolated from Salsola Richteri. TIQs with a 1-methyl substituent occur also in Cactus species. Extensive reviews covering the isoquinoline alkaloids research have been published (Rommelspacher and Susilo, 1985). In bananas acetaldehyde may be enzymatically generated from ethanol produced SAL during the postclimateric phase in the ripening process via the Pictet-Spengler reaction (Riggin et al., 1976). SAL has been measured in various foods and beverages, not only in bananas, but also in soy sauce, wine and beer (Strolin Benedetti et al., 1989a; Duncan and Smythe, 1982; Smythe and Duncan, 1985). These findings suggested that the intake of SAL via dietary sources might affect SAL levels in tissues (Strolin Benedetti et al., 1989b). It was shown that the (R)-enantiomer of SAL predominates in the urine of healthy volunteers ((R/S) ratios between 2.5 and 3.7), whereas the (S)-enantiomer predominates in port wine ((R/S) ratio between 0.3 and 0.35) and possibly in other beverages and foods, suggesting that SAL present in humans could have, at least partially, an endogenous enzymatic origin (Dostert et al., 1987).

In human beeings SAL was first detected in the urine of parkinsonian patients on L-dopa medication (Sandler et al., 1973). Later on, SAL was found in the human brain (Sjöquist et al., 1982; Sasaoka et al., 1988), urine and cerebrospinal fluid (CSF) (Sjöquist et al., 1981a,b). SAL was increased in the urine and in CSF of alcoholics (Collins et al., 1979), and in the urine of patients with phenylketonuria (Lasala and Coscia, 1979).

2.2. Effects of salsolinol

SAL was demonstrated to have a variety of neuropharmacological effects, e.g. it inhibits the uptake of catecholamines, causes the release of stored catecholamines, and is an inhibitor of monoamine oxidase (MAO), catechol-O-methyltransferase (COMT) and tyrosine hydroxylase (Collins et al., 1973; Heikkila et al., 1971; Meyerson et al., 1976; Minami et al., 1992,1993; Weiner and Collins, 1978). When infused directly into the cerebral ventricles of rats, SAL and tetrahydropapaveroline (THP) can enhance markedly the consumption of alcohol (Myers and Melchior, 1977) and they might act centrally to promote a mechanism controlling alcohol drinking.

2.3. Parkinsonism caused by tetrahydroisoquinolines

Administration of TIQs produced remarkable motor disturbances similar to parkinsonism and it is assumed that they might be endogenous substances inducing parkinsonism because of the structural similarity to 1-methyl-4-phenyl-1,2,3,6-tetrahydropyridine (MPTP), an artificial contaminant of illegal meperidine analogue synthesis (Nagatsu and Yoshida, 1988). MPTP is well known to cause parkinsonism in humans with selective neurotoxicity to dopamine neurones in the substantia nigra (Burns et al., 1983; Langston et al., 1983). It is oxidized by type B MAO into a potent neurotoxin, 1-methyl-4-phenylpyridinium ion (MPP+) (Chiba et al., 1984). MPP+ is taken up into cells by the dopamine transport system and this process determines the selectivity of this toxin to dopamine neurons. The cell death of dopamine neurons may be induced by the generation of oxygen radicals, the inhibition of mitochondrial ATP synthesis, or by the induction of apoptotic processes. As candidates of naturally-occuring MPTP-like compounds tetrahydroisoquinolines have been proposed (Nagatsu, 1997; Naoi et al., 1995a). Two reactions, N-methylation and oxidation, produce the N-methylated derivatives and from there the toxic N-methylated cations. Especially, the dopamine-derived tetrahydroisoquinolines are considered as possible candidates (Figure 3).

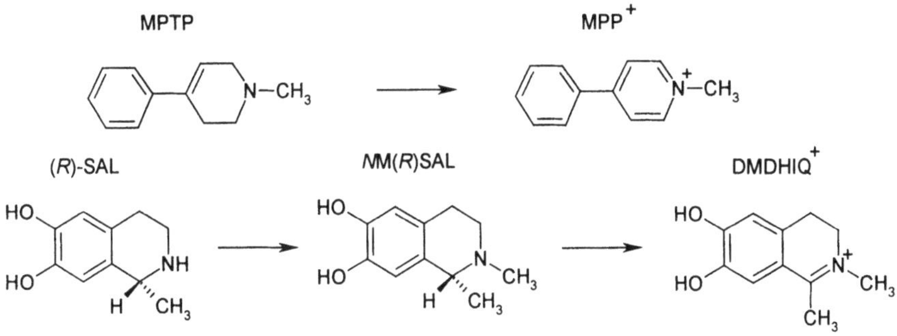

Figure 3 Chemical structures of salsolinol, 1-methyl-4-phenyl-1,2,3,6-tetrahydropyridine (MPTP) and 1-methyl-4-phenylpyridinium ion (MPP+). (R)-Salsolinol is metabolized by a N-methyltransferase into N-methyl(R)-salsolinol (NM(R)SAL) and oxidized into 1,2-dimethyl-6,7-dihydroxyisoquinolinium ion (DMDHIQ+).

2.4. Cytotoxicity of salsolinol

It has been reported that MPP+ inhibits complex I activity (Mizuno et al., 1987a) and adenosine triphosphate (ATP) in the mouse brain (Mizuno et al., 1987b) and mitochondrial respiratory failure, secondary to complex I inhibition, may contribute to the neurodegenerative process underlying nigral cell death. The effects of 22 isoquinoline derivatives on the enzymes of the respiratory chain in mitochondrial fragments of rat forebrain were examined (McNaught et al., 1995b). All compounds inhibited complex I and lipophilicity appeared to be important for inhibition. Furthermore an inhibition of the α-ketoglutarate dehydrogenase complex of the TCA cycle was demonstrated (McNaught et al., 1995a). These findings may represent an additional mechanism contributing to mitochondrial dysfunctions and cell death.

Additionally it was suggested that oxidative stress such as dopamine auto-oxidation and hydroxyl radical generation may be involved in dopamine cell death in normal aging and parkinsonism (Chiueh et al., 1993). NM(R)SAL was found to be oxidized into DMDHIQ+ with concominant formation of hydroxyl radicals. The oxidation and the radical production were completely inhibited by antioxidants, such as ascorbic acid and reduced glutathione, and the radical formation was enhanced by Fe (II) and, to a lesser extent, by Fe (III) in vitro (Maruyama et al., 1995b). A possible mechanism of the selective neurotoxicity of NM(R)SAL to dopaminergic neurons is summarized in figure 4. Using human dopaminergic neuroblastoma SH-SY5Y cells, only NM(R)SAL was found to be accumulated in the cells by the dopamine transport system, but not the (S)-enantiomer of NMSAL (Takahashi et al., 1994). In a rat model it was demonstrated that NM(R)SAL was transported by retrograde axonal flow to cell body into the substantia nigra, oxidized into DMDHIQ+ and accumulated, as shown by analysis of the rat brain regions. Recently, NM(R)SAL and DMDHIQ+ were found to accumulate in the nigro-striatal system in the human brain (Maruyama et al., 1997).

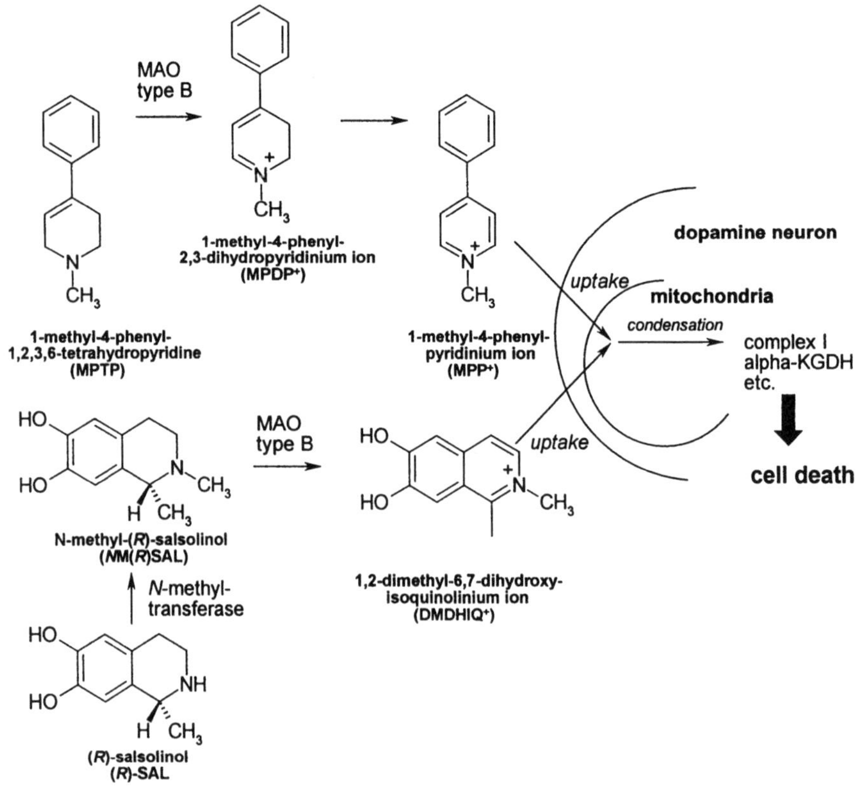

Figure 4 Metabolism of MPTP and SAL in the brain.

This catechol isoquinolinium ion is more cytotoxic than the reduced isoquinoline (Naoi et al., 1996a). Oxidation of NM(R)SAL simultaneously produces hydroxyl radicals, as shown by in vivo (Maruyama et al., 1995a) and in vitro studies (Maruyama et al., 1995b).

The question about the penetration of TIQs into the brain through the blood-brain area is controversial. On the one side there is the hypothesis that SAL cannot be transported into the brain through the blood-brain barrier, so that the SAL detected in the brain requires in situ generation (Origitano and Collins, 1984). However, others showed that the TIQs may be able to penetrate the blood-brain barrier and to accumulate in the brain (Sjöquist and Magnuson, 1980; Kikuchi et al., 1991). Recently, the cytotoxic effects of salsolinol in endothelial cells, which are a major component in the blood-brain barrier, were investigated (Melzig et al., 1998). (S)-SAL was more toxic than the (R)-enantiomer, and the mitochondria were especially a target of the enantioselective toxic effects. The injury of the endothelial cells by SAL might be an indication of a disturbance of the general barrier function. The disturbance of the specific blood-brain barrier by SAL can be followed by an increase in the SAL concentration within the brain, which may then result in toxic effects on neuronal structures leading to patthological effects. To decide whether the cytotoxicity of SAL for endothelial cells was based on its endothelial-specific metabolism, two additional cell lines were used to estimate the cytotoxicity of SAL. In human neuroblastoma cells SK-N-SH as well as in the endocrine line AtT-20/D16v from the anterior pituitary of the mouse the (S)-enantiomer of SAL was more toxic than (R)-SAL. Dopamine itself was less cytotoxic than (S)-SAL, but was in the same range as the (R)-enantiomer. This findings suggested the hypothesis that the (S)-SAL cytotoxicity is induced by a specific, not dopamine receptor mediated mechanism, whereas (R)-SAL had only a nonspecific toxic effect, like dopamine.

2.5. Interaction of salsolinol with dopamine receptors

Alcohol itself does not have any affinity for neuronal receptors of the brain (Myers, 1989), but SAL showed binding to dopamine receptor (Melzig et al., 1998). (S)-SAL showed an affinity to the known five dopamine receptor subtypes, especially to D1- and D3-receptors. With exception of the D3-receptor, the (R)-enantiomer did not show a significant binding to the dopamine receptors. In combination with the fact that SAL induced voluntary alcohol drinking (Myers, 1989) after intracerebroventricular application in rats and the binding of SAL to dopamine receptors, a hypothesis was suggested that SAL is implicated in the production of a β-endorphin deficiency, reported after chronic alcohol consumption (Dave et al., 1986; Seizinger et al., 1984). Additionally, the β-endorphin levels measured in the cerebrospinal fluid of alcoholics were significantly lower than those of controls, whereas the adrenocorticotropin (ACTH) levels were 5 times higher than those of the control values (Genazzani et al., 1982). β-Endorphin and ACTH are important elements of the hypothalamus-pituitary-adrenal stress axis, which is included in the regulation of the reward system and mental processes, like motivation or craving. β-Endorphin and ACTH are formed by limited proteolysis from their precursor peptide proopiomelanocortin (POMC).

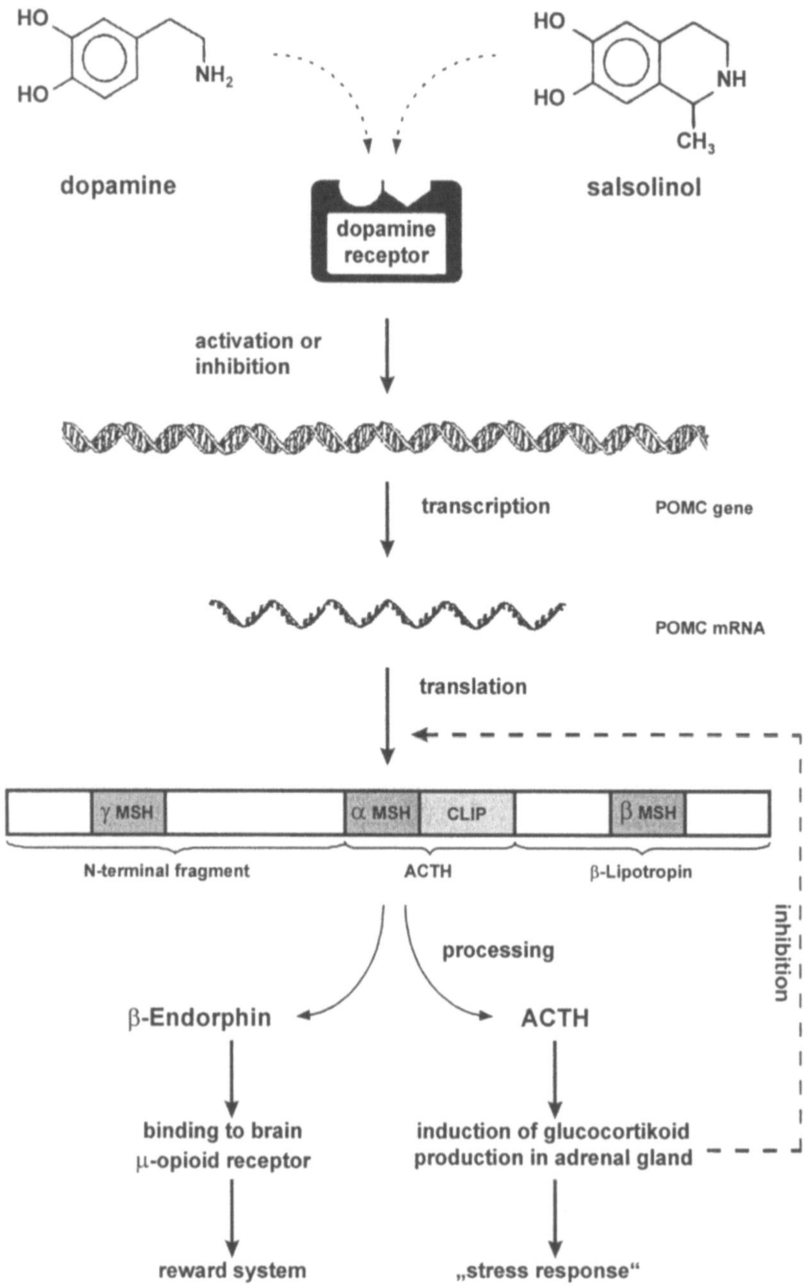

Figure 5 Proposed model for the explanation of the biological effect of SAL in vivo via interaction with dopamine receptors, resulting in changes of the POMC gene expression and inhibited formation of β-endorphin. Modified according toMelzig et al. (1998). (POMC = proopiomelanocortin; ACTH = adrenocorticotropin; MSH = melanocyte-stimulating hormone; CLP = corticotropin-like intermediate peptide).

In experiments with voluntarily alcohol drinking rats the POMC gene expression was dereased after alcohol consumption (Winkler et al., 1995). Recently it was shown that the (S)-enantiomer of SAL caused a significant decrease in the POMC mRNA level (Melzig et al., 1998). Only the intact SAL molecule and not a newly-formed oxidation product was able to inhibit β-endorphin secretion and the secretion process itself was not affected by SAL, but rather the biosynthesis of β-endorphin via the POMC gene expression was. The enantioselectivity of the inhibition of POMC gene expression and β-endorphin secretion by (S)-SAL and the known specific binding of this enantiomer to dopamine receptors are discussed to be strong indications of a link between the chronic effects of alcohol intake and this alkaloid, which might be involved in the establishment of the opioid deficiency in alcoholics via inhibition of POMC gene expression (Figure 5). The stress response is modified via an impaired biosynthesis of ACTH. This changed interaction between the reward system and the stress response as a result of the action of salsolinol seemed to be an important element for the explanation of pharmacological and toxicological effects induced by TIQs.

2.6. Methods for identification and measurement of salsolinol

There are two major methods to detect dopamine-derived TIQ derivatives in tissue (brain) homogenates, CSF, plasma and urine samples. Gas chromatography coupled with mass spectrometry (GC/MS) is the most sensitive and specific method, while the handling of high performance liquid chromatoraphy with electrochemical detection (HPLC/ECD) is easier to perform (Figure 6). Since hydroxylated TIQs are probably in part conjugated, acid hydrolysis or hydrolysis with arylsulfatase and β-glucuronidase should be performed prior to analysis of urine or plasma samples. For the extraction of catecholic TIQs from biological samples, such cleanup procedures for catecholamine detection, as absorption on alumina combined with solid-phase extraction, are usually used. For a selective solid-phase extraction, especially from urine or plasma samples, a phenylboronic acid sorbent is useful. Brain tissue with a high content of lipids can be used after incubation with lipase prior to extraction. The identification of the two enantiomers of SAL was first achieved by GC and nitrogen-phophorous detection after methylation with diazomethane and then derivatization to the diastereomers with N-trifluoroacetyl-L-prolyl chloride (Dostert et al., 1987). Later on, a HPLC procedure was developed with the same derivatization method (Strolin Benedetti et al., 1989a,b). Then, this method was modified by using a chiral derivatizing agent, (S)-1-(1-naphthyl)ethyl isothiocyanate, and a good resolution of the two diastereomers was obtained (Pianezzola et al., 1989). Today for the HPLC determination (R/S)-SAL are separated using a β-cyclodextrin-OH phase column or using β-cyclodextrin in a reversed-phase ion-pair system. The eluate is monitored electrochemically, without further preparation or derivatization (Sällström Baum and Rommelspacher, 1994; Deng et al., 1995, 1996, 1997). In our opinion a sensitive and reliable gas chromatographic method is more useful for the determination of SAL enantiomers. Using GC/MS, not only peak detection but also peak identification is achieved. (R/S)-SAL are transformed into diastereomers by a two-step derivatization with N-methyl-N-trimethylsilyltrifluoracetamide (MSTFA) and (R)-(-)-2-phenyl butyryl chloride as a chiral derivatization agent, which reveals baseline-resolved peaks on a conventional GC column (Haber et al., 1995a; Musshoff et al., 2000). In figures 7 and 8 the electron mass spectra of dopamine, salsolinol and norsalsolinol after derivatization are described together with a gas chromatogram (EI-SIM) of a spiked brain sample. Obtaining high specificity is the major consideration using GC/MS, because HPLC methods, even in conjunction with electrochemical detection, are not sufficiently specific to allow selective detection and quantification of SAL enantiomers. In biological matrices, co-extraction of unknown compounds can lead to a complex chromatogram and often to overlaps between analytes and interfering peaks.

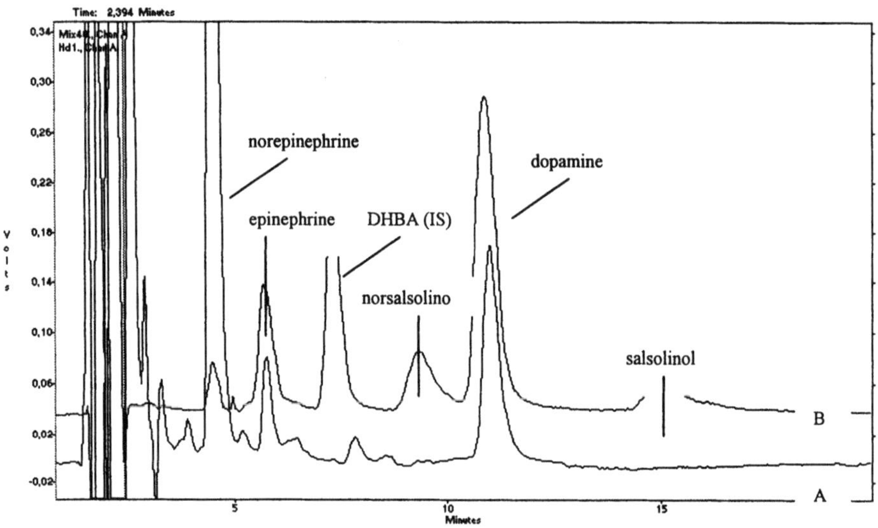

Figure 6 HPLC chromatograms of authentic human brain sample extracts. A: Frontal cortex without additon of the internal standard (DHBA = 3,4-dihydroxybenzylamine). B: Example for an extract of the hypothalamus containing epinephrine, norepinephrine and dopamine, norsalsolinol and salsolinol (Musshoff et al., 1999)

3. Alcoholism and Salsolinol

Although the involvement of TIQs in the brain function has been demonstrated in many experiments, the concrete evidence for their formation in elevated concentrations after alcohol abuse is still lacking. Conflicting results were reported on the change of SAL levels after alcohol ingestion. SAL was significantly elevated in urine samples from alcoholics at the first day of admission for detoxification and dropped to control excretion values after several days (Collins et al., 1979). Others have confirmed elevated urine SAL levels at administration but no significant decrease in these levels at 3 weeks postwithdrawal (Sjöquist et al., 1981a). In contrast, little difference from controls for admission day SAL levels were reported in alcoholics, during early detoxification, a tendency towards increased excretion was observed in other studies (Clow et al., 1985; Feest et al., 1992).

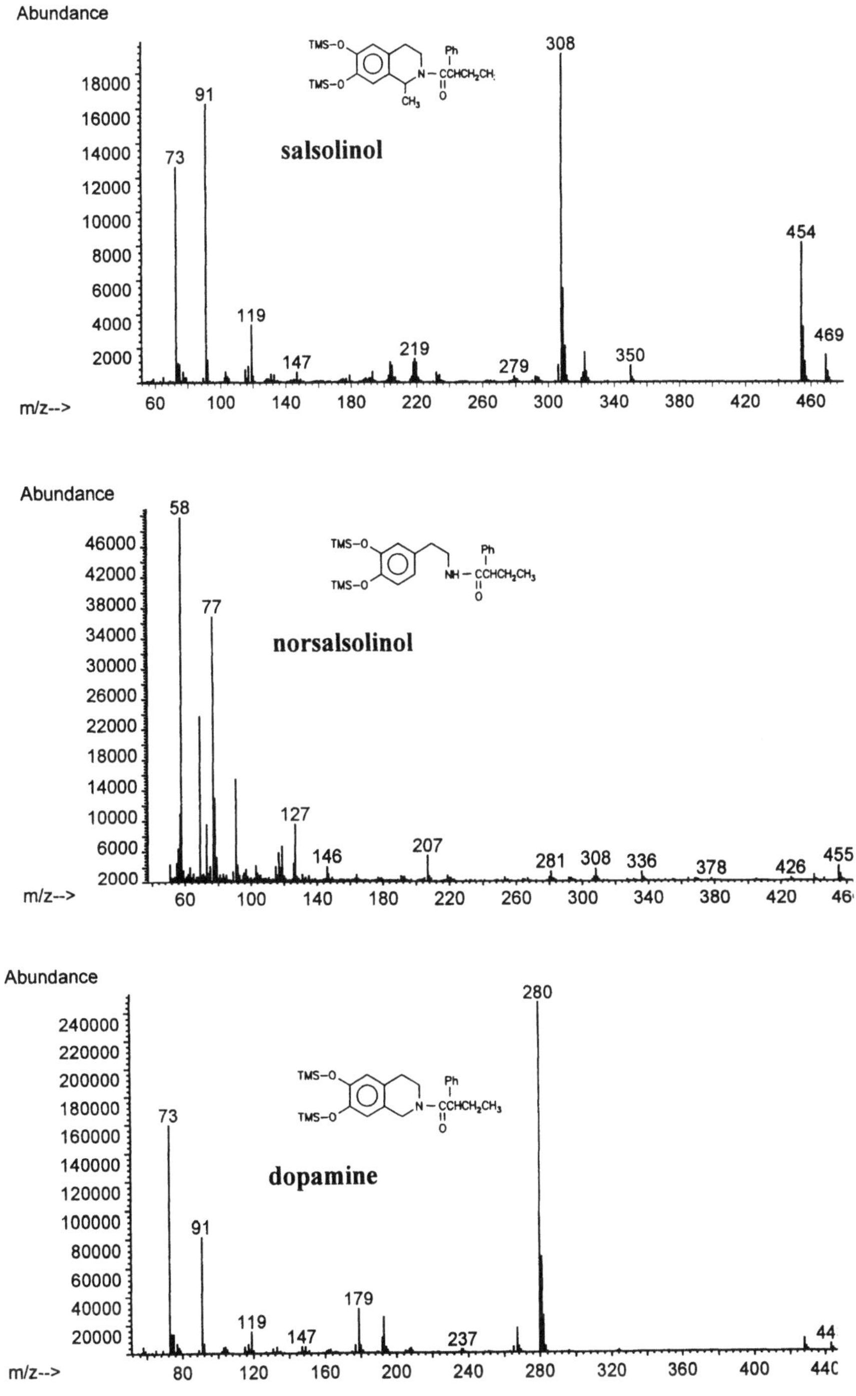

Figures 7 Electron-impact (EI) mass spectra of dopamine, salsolinol and norsalsolinol after a two-step derivatization with MSTFA and (R)-(-)-2-phenylbutyryl chloride (Musshoff et al., 2000)

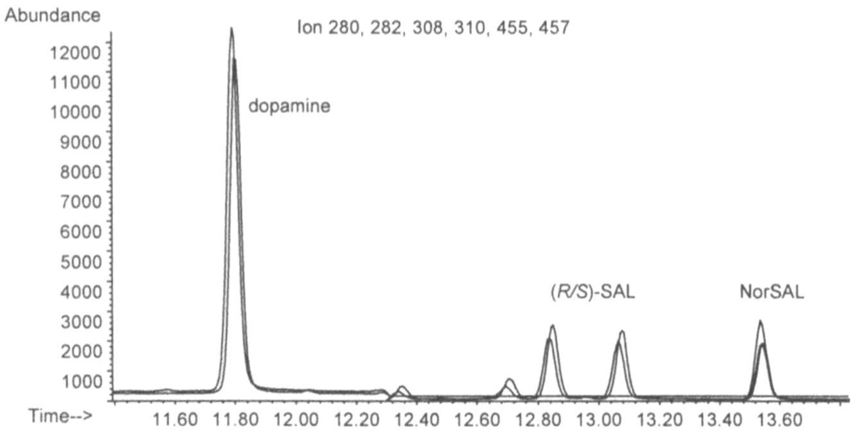

Figure 8 Gas chromatogram (EI-SIM) of a spiked brain sample assyed to contain 25 ng of (R/S)-SAL and NorSAL and 250 ng of dopamie (Musshoff et al., 200))

However, due to great interindividual variations both the urinary SAL level and the SAL excretion rate are insufficient markers to distinguish between alcoholics and nonalcoholics. Otherwise, using the concentration ratio of NorSAL and SAL (dopamine-aldehyde adduct ratio; DAAR), significantly higher ratios were observed in alcoholics (median 1.3) compared with non-alcoholics (median 0.6) ($p = 0.0001$; Wilcoxon signed-rank sum at 5 % level) (Musshoff et al., 1996, 1997).

The DAAR could be an indicator of metabolic stress or metabolic derailment. A displacement toward NorSAL can be seen under the influence of ingested/accumulated methanol on the C1 metabolism, producing increased formation of formaldehyde condensation products. The DAAR could also indicate an increased dopamine level in manifestly sick persons. Because formaldehyde is 15 times as reactive as acetaldehyde in the Pictet-Spengler reaction with dopamine, the level of NorSAL is increased based on the higher availability of the educt dopamine, particulary during withdrawal, when the levels of methanol and formaldehyde are increased significantly.

Elevated concentrations of SAL sulfate have been determined in blood plasma of alcoholics during the 3-30 days withdrawal period (Faraj et al., 1989). In further studies it has been demonstrated that (R)-SAL predominates in human urine (Strolin Benedetti et al., 1989a). The (S)-enantiomer seemed to be formed in individuals who drink substantial amounts of alcoholic beverages regularly over a period of time and it has been speculated that ethanol-derived acetaldehyde favors the production of racemic SAL explaining elevated (R)- and (S)-SAL levels (Dostert et al., 1988, 1991). It has been shown that the urinary SAL output and the SAL levels in plasma are significantly influenced by the intake of ethanol (Haber et al., 1995b, 1996; Rommelspacher et al., 1995). The different changes of the

SAL output are discussed to be affected by a genetic predisposition for an alcohol-induced SAL formation.

The variability in the reported data might be a result of variables including dietary conditions during the experiments or the duration of ethanol ingestion and analytical problems associated with the detectability of the TIQs.

In the research of the pathogenesis of parkinsonism the enantio-specific occurence of only (R)-SAL and N-methyl-(R)-salsolinol (NM(R)-SAL) in cerebrospinal fluid (CSF) (Maruyama et al., 1996a), intraventricular fluid (Maruyama et al., 1996b), and in the human brain (Maruyama et al., 1997) suggested their enzymatic synthesis in the human brain by two steps: synthesis of (R)-SAL by a salsolinol synthase (Naoi et al., 1996b), and N-methylation by a N-methyltransferase (Naoi et al., 1997). NM(R)SAL was found to be oxidized enzymatically (Naoi et al., 1995b) and non-enzymatically (Maruyama et al., 1995b) into the cytotoxic 1,2-dimethyl-6,7-dihydroxyisoquinolinium ion (DMDHIQ+). An ubiquitous distribution of (R)-SAL (and the salsolinol synthase) was reported in the brain, the (S)-enantiomer was not detected in any brain region. On the other hand, NM(R)SAL and

DMDHIQ+ were found to accumulate in the nigro-striatal system, which was explained to higher activity of a N-methyltransferase in the substantia nigra.

We carried out a systematic regional study of dopamine and dopamine-derived salsolinol and norsalsolinol levels in human brain areas (Musshoff et al., 1999). In figure 9 (p.128) the distribution of the main central neuronal pathways containing dopamine are demonstrated. Dopamine concentrations determined by high performance liquid chromatography coupled with electrochemical detection (HPLC/ECD) were highest in the basal ganglia, especially in the striatum (putamen and nucleus caudatus-accumbens), followed by the substantia nigra and the hypothalamus (Table 1).

n = 32	dopamine (ng/g ± S.D.)	salsolinol (ng/g ± S.D.)	norsalsolinol (ng/g ± S.D.)
Basal ganglia			
Nucl. Accumbens	986 ± 435.3	43.1 ± 33.7	45.1 ± 43.9
Nucl. Caudatus	2470 ± 828.6	38.5 ± 35.3	50.4 ± 43.7
Putamen	1170 ± 450.8	35.1 ± 30.7	25.,1 ± 30.7
Subst. Nigra	384 ± 131.6	5.1 ± 3.7	8.1 ± 7.7
Hypothalamus	186 ± 134.9	0.5 ± 1.1	0.6 ± 0.8
Med. oblongata	102 ± 80.5	-	-

n = 32	dopamine (ng/g ± S.D.)	salsolinol (ng/g ± S.D.)	norsalsolinol (ng/g ± S.D.)
Thalamus	43 ± 18.9	-	-
Nuc. Amygdalis	20 ± 7.7	-	-
Frontal cortex	19 ± 10.0	-	-
Gyrus precentralis	15 ± 12.,1	-	-
Nucl. tegment.	12 ± 9.9	-	-
Hippocampus	11 ± 3.9	-	-
Tub. olfact.	11 ± 8.9	-	-
White Matter	10 ± 10.1	-	-
Cerebellum	8 ± 6.0	-	-

Table 1 Levels of dopamine, salsolinol and norsalsolinol in various human brain areas determined using HPLC with electrochemical detection (Musshoff et al., 1999).

In all brain areas measurable amounts of dopamine were found. Low concentrations were detected in the white matter, cerebellum, hippocampus, frontal cortex, amygdaloid nucleus and thalamus. Significant amounts of SAL and NorSAL were found in the dopamine-rich areas, the striatum, substantia nigra and hypothalamus. In other regions there was no evidence for these alkaloids. These findings suggested that the concentration of the substrate dopamine may determine the level of SAL during in vivo formation. However, we demonstrated the formation of SAL and NorSAL in those brain areas, which are responsible for addiction processes.In a further study using a solid-phase extraction procedure and a gas chromatographic - mass spectrometric method including a two-step derivatization with MSTFA and (R)-(-)-2-phenylbutyryl chloride high resolution of (R/S)-salsolinol was achieved after transforming into diastereomers (Musshoff et al., 2000). The objective was to evaluate differences of stereospecific synthesis of SAL and a possible relationship between brain levels of dopamine and (R/S)-SAL or NorSAL in the most relevant brain areas. We detected dopamine, NorSAL and both SAL enantiomers (Table 2).

n = 25	Dopamine (ng/g ± S.D.)	(*R*)-salsolinol (ng/g ± S.D.)	(*S*)-salsolinol (ng/g ± S.D.)	norsalsolinol (ng/g ± S.D.)
Nucl. accumbens	622 ± 485	16.5 ± 6.3	7.8 ± 6.1	55.5 ± 28.9
Nucl. caudatus	1905 ± 975	12.5 ± 8.9	7.9 ± 6.3	42.1 ± 37.8
Putamen	1055 ± 622	24.1 ± 20.9	14.2 ± 12.0	40.0 ± 20.3
Subst. nigra	285 ± 236	28.6 ± 18.3	18.5 ± 14.1	12.3 ± 9.2
Hypothalamus	155 ± 123	11.9 ± 9.8	12.8 ± 10.8	4.5 ± 2.8

Table 2 Dopamine and dopamine-derived (R/S)-salsolinol and norsalsolinol levels determined in various human brain areas using GC/MS (Musshoff et al., 2000).

However, (R)-SAL was found to be predominant with a (R)-/(S)-SAL ratio of approximately 2 in all brain regions. These findings did not support the hypothesis that only an enantio-selective synthesis of (R)-SAL by a putative salsolinol synthase is responsible for the in vivo formation. Furthermore, the missing correlations between levels of (R)-SAL, (S)-SAL, and dopamine do not further strengthen the concept of an exclusive enzymatic synthesis. Our findings are in accordance with Müller et al. (1999), who also found (R)-SAL and (S)-SAL in plasma and CSF in parkinsonian subjects or control subjects with no association of dopamine levels with SAL levels. However, the detection of (S)-SAL does not exclude an enzymatic pathway for the endogenous SAL formation. In our opinion a non-enzymatic formation of SAL via Pictet-Spengler reaction could result in both, (R)- and (S)-SAL, and an additional enzymatic synthesis of only (R)-SAL could explain the enantiomer ratio (R)-/(S)-SAL of approximately 2. Also an alcohol-induced enzymatic formation of (S)-SAL could be possible. The described increased levels of NM(R)-SAL may be caused by upregulation of N-methyltransferase specific for (R)-SAL.

The variability in the reported data (see the standard deviations, which are described also by other authors) might be a result of variables including dietary conditi ons, the duration of ethanol ingestion or might be influenced by neurologic or psychiatric illness or other factors. These variables have to be taken into account for further investigations.

4. Further investigatons

To further clarify the biosynthesis and the origin of brain SAL and NorSAL it is mandatory to determine the stereoisomers of SAL in the brain of subjects with known histories of alcoholism and of neurologic or neurogenerative disorders. Our recent results indicate an age-dependent decrease in the dopamine and SAL levels, which may be ascribed to the decrease of dopamine neurons and dopamine synthesis by aging. Further investigations could be helpful for the understanding of the etiology of diseases involving dopamine-derived tetrahydroisoquinolines.

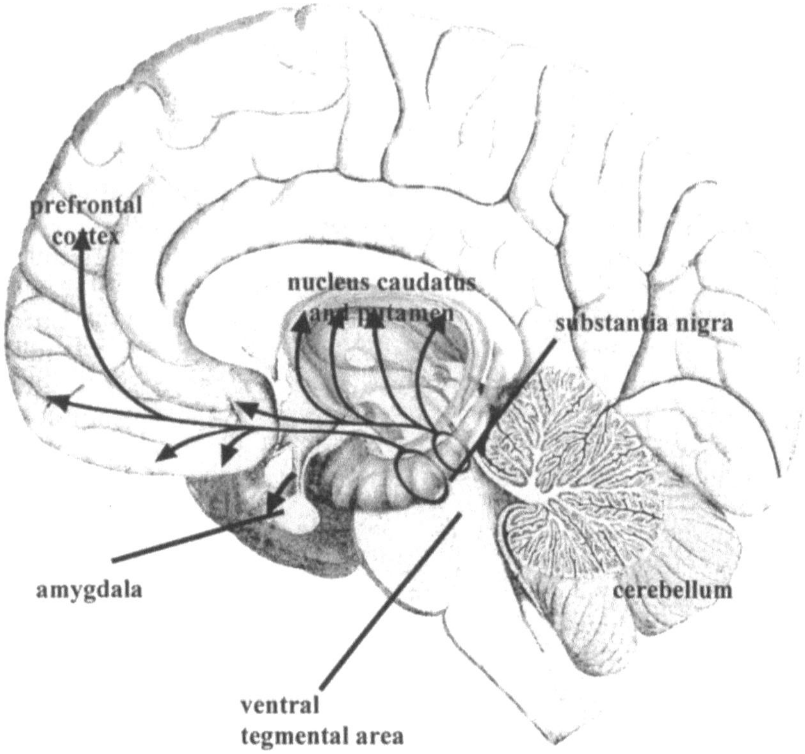

Figure 9 Schematic demonstration illustrating the distribution of the main central neuronal pathways containing dopamine.

Acknowledgements

The brain studies were supported by the BONFOR-Forschungskommission, Bonn, Germany (No. 148/02).

References

Brossi A. (1982) Mammalian TIQ's: products of condensation with aldehydes or pyruvic acids? Prog. Clin. Biol. Res., 90, 125-133.

Burns R.S., Chiueh C.C., Markey S.P., Ebert M.H., Jacobowitz D.M. and Kopin I.J. (1983) A primate model of parkinsonism:selective destruction of dopaminergic neurons in the pars compacta of substantia nigra by N-methyl-4-phenyl-1,2,3,6-tetrahydropyridine. Proc. Natl. Acad. Sci.USA, 80, 4546-4550.

Chiba K., Trevor A.J. and Castagnoli N. (1984) Metabolism of the neurotoxic amine, MPTP, by brain monoamine oxidase. Biochem. Biphys. Res. Commun., 120, 574-578.

Chiueh C.C., Miyake H. and Peng M.-T. (1993) Role of dopamine autooxidation, hydroxyl radical generation, and calcium overload in underlying mechanisms involved in MPTP-induced parkinsonism. Adv. Neurol., 60, 251-258.

Clow A., Topham A., Saunders J.B., Murray R. and Sandler M. (1985) The role of salsolinol in alcohol intake and withdrawal. Prog. Clin. Biol. Res., 183, 101-113.

Cohen G. and Collins M. (1970) Alkaloids from catecholamines in adrenal tissue: Possible role in alcoholism. Science, 167, 1749-1751.

Collins A.C., Cashaw J.L. and Davis V.E. (1973) Dopamine-derived tetrahydroisoquinoline alkaloids - inhibitors of neuroamine metabolism. Biochem. Pharmacol., 22, 2337-2348.

Collins M.A., Nijm W.P., Borge G.F., Teas G. and Goldfarb C. (1979) Dopamine-related tetrahydroisoquinolines: significant urinary excretion by alcoholics after alcohol consumption. Science, 206, 1184-1186.

Dave J.R., Lee E.E., Karanian J.W. and Eskay R.L. (1986) Ethanol exposure decreases pituitary corticotrophin-releasing factor binding, adenylate cyclase activity, proopiomelanocortin biosynthesis and plasma ß-endorphin. Endocrinology, 118, 280-286.

Davis V.E. and Walsh M.J. (1970) Alcohol, amines, and alkaloids: A possible biochemical basis for alcohol addiction. Science, 167, 1005-1007.

Deng Y., Maruyama W., Dostert P., Takahashi T., Kawai M. and Naoi M. (1995) Determination of the (R)- and (S)-enantiomers of salsolinol and N-methylsalsolinol by use of a chiral high-performance liquid chromatographic column. J. Chromatogr. B, 670, 47-54.

Deng Y., Maruyama W., Kawai M., Dostert P., Yamamura H., Takahashi T. and Naoi M. (1997) Assay for the (R)- and (S)-enantiomers of salsolinols in biological samples and foods with ion-pair high-performance liquid chromatography using beta-cyclodextrin as a chiral mobile phase additive. J. Chromatogr. B, 689, 313-320.

Deng Y., Maruyama W., Yamamura H., Kawai M., Dostert P. and Naoi M. (1996) Mechanism of enantioseparation of salsolinols, endogenous neurotoxins in human brain, with ion-pair chromatography using beta-cyclodextrin as a mobile phase additive. Anal. Chem., 68, 2826-2831.

Dostert P., Strolin Benedetti M. and Dedieu M. (1987) Ratio of enantiomers of salsolinol in human urine. Pharmacol. Toxicol., 60 [Suppl. 1], 13.

Dostert P., Strolin Benedetti M. and Dordain G. (1988) Dopamine-derived alkaloids in alcoholism and in Parkinson's and Huntington's diseases. J. Neural Transm., 74, 61-74.

Dostert P., Strolin Benedetti M., Dordain G. and Vernay D. (1991) Urinary elimination of salsolinol enantiomers in alcoholics. J. Neural Transm., 85, 51-59.

Duncan M.W. and Smythe G.A. (1982) Salsolinol and dopamine in alcoholic beverages [letter]. Lancet, 1, 904-905.

Faraj B.A., Camp V.M., Davis D.C., Lenton J.D. and Kutner M. (1989) Elevation of plasma salsolinol sulfate in chronic alcoholics as compared to nonalcoholics. Alcohol Clin. Exp. Res., 13, 155-163.

Feest U., Kemper A., Nickel B., Rabe H. and Koalick F. (1992) Comparison of salsolinol excretion in alcoholics and nonalcoholic controls. Alcohol, 9, 49-52.

Genazzani A.R., Nappi G., Facchinetti G.L., Mazella G.L., Petraglia F. and Savoldi F. (1982) Central deficiency of beta-endorphine in alcohol addicts. Clin. Endocrinol. Metab., 55, 583-586.

Haber H. and Melzig M. (1992) [Tetrahydroisoquinolines - endogenous products from chronic alcohol abuse]. Pharmazie, 47, 3-7.

Haber H., Henklein P., Georgi M. and Melzig M.F. (1995a) Resolution of catecholic tetrahydroisoquinoline enantiomers and the determination of R- and S-salsolinol in biological samples by gas chromatography-mass spectrometry. J. Chromatogr.B, 672, 179-187.

Haber H., Putscher I., Georgi M. and Melzig M.F. (1995b) Influence of ethanol on the salsolinol excretion in healthy subjects. Alcohol, 12, 299-303.

Haber H., Winkler A., Putscher I., Henklein P., Baeger I., Georgi M. and Melzig M.F. (1996) Plasma and urine salsolinol in humans: effect of acute ethanol intake on the enantiomeric composition of salsolinol. Alcohol Clin. Exp. Res., 20, 87-92.

Heikkila R., Cohen G. and Dembiec D. (1971) Tetrahydroisoquinoline alkaloids: uptake by rat brain homogenates and inhibition of catecholamine uptake. Pharmacol. Exp. Ther., 179, 250-258.

Kajita M., Niwa T., Maruyama W., Nakahara D., Takeda N., Yoshizumi H., Tatematsu A., Watanabe K., Naoi M. and Nagatsu T. (1994) Endogenous synthesis of N-methylnorsalsolinol in rat brain during in vivo microdialysis with epinine. J. Chromatogr. B, 654, 263-269.

Kikuchi K., Nagatsu Y., Makino Y., Mashino T., Ohta S. and Hirobe M. (1991) Metabolism and penetration through blood-brain barrier of parkinsonism-related compounds. 1,2,3,4-Tetrahydroisoquinoline and 1-methyl-1,2,3,4-tetrahydroisoquinoline. Drug Metab. Dispos., 19, 257-262.

Langston J.W., Ballard P., Tetrud J.W. and Irwin I. (1983) Chronic parkinsonism in humans due to a product of meperidine-analog synthesis. Science, 219, 979-980.

Lasala J.M. and Coscia C.J. (1979) Accumulation of a tetrahydroisoquinoline in phenylketonuria. Science, 203, 283-284.

Maruyama W., Abr T., Toghi H., Dostert P. and Naoi M. (1996a) A dopaminergic neurotoxin, (R)-N-methylsalsolinol, increases in parkinsonian CSF. Ann. Neurol., 40, 119-122.

Maruyama W., Dostert P. and Naoi M. (1995a) Dopamine-derived 1-methyl-6,7-dihydroxyisoquinolines as hydroxyl radical promoters and scavengers in the rat brain: in vivo and in vitro studies. J. Neurochem., 64, 2635-2643.

Maruyama W., Dostert P., Matsubara K. and Naoi, M. (1995b) N-methyl(R)salsolinol produces hydroxyl radicals: involvement to neurotoxicity. Free Radic. Biol. Med., 19, 67-75.

Maruyama W., Nakahara D., Ota M., Takahashi T., Takahashi A., Nagatsu T. and Naoi M. (1992) N-methylation of dopamine-derived 6,7-dihydroxy-1,2,3,4- tetrahydroisoquinoline, (R)-salsolinol, in rat brains: in vivo microdialysis study. J. Neurochem., 59, 395-400.

Maruyama W., Narabayashi H., Dostert P. and Naoi M. (1996b) Stereospecific occurrence of a parkinsonism-inducing catechol isoquinoline, N-methyl(R)salsolinol, in the human intraventricular fluid. J. Neural Transm., 103, 1069-1076.

Maruyama W., Sobue G., Matsubara K., Hashizume Y., Dostert P. and Naoi M. (1997) A dopaminergic neurotoxin, 1(R), 2(N)-dimethyl-6,7-dihydroxy-1,2, 3,4-tetrahydroisoquinoline, N-methyl(R)salsolinol, and its oxidation product, 1,2(N)-dimethyl-6,7-dihydroxyisoquinolinium ion, accumulate in the nigro-striatal system of the human brain. Neurosci. Lett., 223, 61-64.

McNaught K.S., Altomare C., Cellamare S., Carotti A., Thull U., Carrupt P.A., Testa B., Jenner P. and Marsden C.D. (1995a) Inhibition of alpha-ketoglutarate dehydrogenase by isoquinoline derivatives structurally related to 1-methyl-1,2,3,6-tetrahydropyridine (MPTP). Neuroreport, 6, 1105-1108.

McNaught K.S., Thull U., Carrupt P.A., Altomare C., Cellamare S., Carotti A., Testa B., Jenner P. and Marsden C.D. (1995b) Inhibition of complex I by isoquinoline derivatives structurally related to 1-methyl-4-phenyl-1,2,3,6-tetrahydropyridine (MPTP). Biochem. Pharmacol., 50, 1903-1911.

Melzig M.F., Putscher I., Haber H., Rottmann M. and Zipper J. (1998) Toxicity and pharmacological effects of salsolinol in different cultivated cells. In: Moser A. (ed.), Pharmacology of endogenous neurotoxins - a handbook (pp. 253-266). Boston: Birkhaeuser.

Meyerson L.R., McMurtrey K.D. and Davis V.E. (1976) Neuroamine-derived alkaloids: Substrate-preferred inhibitors of rat brain monoamine oxidase in vitro. Biochem. Pharmacol., 25, 1013-1020.

Minami M., Maruyama W., Dostert P., Nagatsu T. and Naoi M. (1993) Inhibition of type A and B monoamine oxidase by 6,7-dihydroxy-1, 2,3,4-tetrahydroisoquinolines and their N-methylated derivatives. J. Neural Transm., 92, 125-135.

Minami M., Takahashi T., Maruyama W., Takahashi A., Dostert P., Nagatsu T. and Naoi M. (1992) Inhibition of tyrosine hydroxylase by R and S enantiomers of salsolinol, 1-methyl-6,7-dihydroxy-1,2,3,4-tetrahydroisoquinoline. J. Neurochem., 58, 2097-2101.

Mizuno Y., Saitoh T. and Sone N. (1987a) Inhibition of mitochondrial NADH-ubiquinone oxidoreductase activity by 1-methyl-4-phenylpyridinium ion. Biochem. Biophys. Res. Commun., 143, 294-299.

Mizuno Y., Suzuki K., Sone N. and Saitoh T. (1987b) Inhibition of ATP synthesis by 1-methyl-4-phenylpyridinium ion (MPP+) in isolated mitochondria from mouse brains. Neurosci. Lett., 81, 204-208.

Müller T., Przuntek H., Kuhn W., Sällström Baum S. and Rommelspacher H. (1999) No increase of synthesis of (R)salsolinol in Parkinson's disease. Mov. Disord., 14, 514-515.

Musshoff F., Daldrup T., Bonte W., Leitner A. and Lesch O.M. (1996) Formaldehyde-derived tetrahydroisoquinolines and tetrahydro-beta- carbolines in human urine. J. Chromatogr. B, 683, 163-176.

Musshoff F., Daldrup T., Bonte W., Leitner A. and Lesch, O.M. (1997) Salsolinol and norsalsolinol in human urine samples. Pharmacol. Biochem. Behav., 58, 545-550.

Musshoff F., Schmidt P., Dettmeyer R., Priemer F., Jachau K. and Madea B. (2000) Determination of dopamine and dopamine-derived (R)-/(S)-salsolinol and norsalsolinol in various human brain areas using solid-phase extraction and gas chromatography / mass spectrometry. Forensic Sci. Int., 113, 356-366.

Musshoff F., Schmidt P., Dettmeyer R., Priemer F., Wittig H. and Madea B. (1999) A systematic study of dopamine and dopamine-derived salsolinol and norsalsolinol levels in human brain areas. Forensic Sci. Int., 105, 1-11.

Myers R.D. (1989) Isoquinolines, beta-carbolines and alcohol drinking: involvement of opioid and dopaminergic mechanisms. Experientia, 45, 436-443.

Myers R.D. and Melchior C.L. (1977) Differential actions on voluntary alcohol intake of tetrahydroisoquinolines or a beta-carboline infused chronically in the ventricle of the rat. Pharmacol. Biochem. Behav., 7, 381-392.

Nagatsu, T. (1997) Isoquinoline neurotoxins in the brain and Parkinson's disease. Neurosci. Res., 29, 99-111.

Nagatsu T. and Yoshida M. (1988) An endogenous substance of the brain, tetrahydroisoquinoline, produces parkinsonism in primates with decreased dopamine, tyrosine hydroxylase and biopterin in the nigrostriatal regions. Neurosci. Lett., 87, 178-182.

Naoi M., Maruyama W. and Dostert P. (1995a) Dopamine-derived 6,7-dihydroxy-1,2,3,4-tetrahydroisoquinolines; oxidation and neurotoxicity. Prog. Brain Res., 106, 227-239.

Naoi M., Maruyama W., Dostert P. and Hashizume Y. (1996a) Animal model of parkinson's disease induced by naturely-occuring 1(R),2(N)-dimethyl-6,7-dihydroxy-1,2,3,4-tetrahydroisoquinoline. Biogenic Amines, 12, 132-147.

Naoi M., Maruyama W., Dostert P., Kohda K. and Kaiya T. (1996b) A novel enzyme enantio-selectively synthesizes (R)salsolinol, a precursor of a dopaminergic neurotoxin, N-methyl(R)salsolinol. Neurosci.Lett., 212, 183-186.

Naoi M., Maruyama W., Matsubara K. and Hashizume Y. (1997) A neutral N-methyltransferase activity in the striatum determines the level of an endogenous MPP+-like neurotoxin, 1,2- dimethyl-6,7-dihydroxyisoquinolinium ion, in the substantia nigra of human brains. Neurosci.Lett., 235, 81-84.

Naoi M., Maruyama W., Zhang J.H., Takahashi T., Deng Y. and Dostert P. (1995b) Enzymatic oxidation of the dopaminergic neurotoxin, 1(R), 2(N)-dimethyl-6,7-dihydroxy-1,2,3,4-tetrahydroisoquinoline, into 1, 2(N)-dimethyl-6,7-dihydroxyisoquinolinium ion. Life Sci., 57, 1061-1066.

Origitano T.C. and Collins M.A. (1984) Gas chromatographic analysis of endogenous catecholamines, phenolic amines and derived isoquinolines using short glass capillary columns and electron-capture detection. J. Chromatogr., 311, 17-29.

Pianezzola E., Bellotti V., Fontana E., Moro E., Gal J. and Desai D.M. (1989) Determination of the enantiomeric composition of salsolinol in biological samples by high-performance liquid chromatography with electrochemical detection. J. Chromatogr., 495, 205-214.

Riggin R.M., McCarthy M.J. and Kissinger, P.T. (1976) Identification of salsolinol as a major dopamine metabolite in the banana. J. Agric. Food Chem., 24, 189-191.

Robbins J.H. (1968) Alkaloid formation by condensation of biogenic amines with acetaldehyde. Clin. Res., 16, 350-350.

Rommelspacher H. and Susilo R. (1985) Tetrahydroisoquinolines and beta-carbolines: putative natural substances in plants and mammals. Prog. Drug Res., 29, 415-459.

Rommelspacher H., Sällstrom Baum S., Dufeu P. and Schmidt L.G. (1995) Determination of (R)- and (S)-salsolinol sulfate and dopamine sulfate levels in plasma of nonalcoholics and alcoholics. Alcohol, 12, 309-315.

Sällström Baum S. and Rommelspacher H. (1994) Determination of total dopamine, R- and S-salsolinol in human plasma by cyclodextrin bonded-phase liquid chromatography with electrochemical detection. J. Chromatogr. B, 660, 235-241.

Sandler M., Carter S.B., Hunter K.R. and Stern G.M. (1973) Tetrahydroisoquinoline alkaloids: in vivo metabolites of L-dopa in man. Nature, 241, 439-443.

Sasaoka T., Kaneda N., Niwa T., Hashizume Y. and Nagatsu T. (1988) Analysis of salsolinol in human brain using high-performance liquid chromatography with electrochemical detection. J. Chromatogr., 428, 152-155.

Seizinger B.R., Höllt V. and Herz A. (1984) Effects of chronic ethanol treatment on the in vitro biosynthesis of pro-opiomelanocortin and its posttranslational processing to beta-endorphin in the intermediate lobe of the rat pituitary. J. Neurochem., 43, 607-613.

Sjöquist B. and Magnuson E. (1980) Analysis of salsolinol and salsoline in biological samples using deuterium-labelled internal standards and gas chromatography - mass spectrometry. J. Chromatogr., 183, 17-24.

Sjöquist B., Borg S. and Kvande H. (1981a) Catecholamine derived compounds in urine and cerebrospinal fluid from alcoholics during and after long-standing intoxication. Subst.Alcohol Actions Misuse., 2, 63-72.

Sjöquist B., Borg S. and Kvande H. (1981b) Salsolinol and methylated salsolinol in urine and cerebrospinal fluid from healthy volunteers. Subst. Alcohol Actions Misuse., 2, 73-77.

Sjöquist B., Eriksson A. and Winblad B. (1982) Salsolinol and catecholamines in human brain and their relation to alcoholism. Prog. Clin. Biol. Res., 90, 57-67.

Smythe G.A. and Duncan M.W. (1985) Precise GC/MS assays for salsolinol and tetrahydropapaveroline: the question of artifacts and dietary sources and the influence of alcohol. Prog. Clin. Biol. Res., 183, 77-84.

Strolin Benedetti M., Bellotti V., Pianezzola E., Moro E., Carminati P. and Dostert P. (1989a) Ratio of the R and S enantiomers of salsolinol in food and human urine. J. Neural Transm., 77, 47-53.

Strolin Benedetti M., Dostert P. and Carminati, P. (1989b) Influence of food intake on the enantiomeric composition of urinary salsolinol in man. J. Neural Transm., 78, 43-51.

Takahashi T., Deng Y., Maruyama W., Dostert P., Kawai M. and Naoi M. (1994) Uptake of a neurotoxin-candidate, (R)-1,2-dimethyl-6,7-dihydroxy-1,2,3,4-tetrahydroisoquinoline into human dopaminergic neuroblastoma SH-SY5Y cells by dopamine transport system. J. Neural Transm., 98, 107-118.

Weiner C. and Collins M. (1978) Tetrahydroisoquinolines derived from catecholamines or dopa: Effects on brain tyrosine hydroxylase activity. Biochem. Pharmacol., 27, 2699-2703.

Winkler A., Roske I., Furkert J., Fickel J. and Melzig M.F. (1995) Effects of voluntary ethanol ingestion on the POMC gene expression in the rat pituitary and on the plasma ß-endorphin content. Alcohol Alcoholism, 30, 231-238.

MIX
Papier aus verantwortungsvollen Quellen
Paper from responsible sources
FSC® C105338

If you have any concerns about our products,
you can contact us on
ProductSafety@springernature.com

In case Publisher is established outside the EU,
the EU authorized representative is:
Springer Nature Customer Service Center GmbH
Europaplatz 3, 69115 Heidelberg, Germany

Printed by Libri Plureos GmbH
in Hamburg, Germany